PEDIATRIC NURSING, PSYCHIATRIC AND SURGICAL ISSUES

Edited by **Öner Özdemir**

Pediatric Nursing, Psychiatric and Surgical Issues
http://dx.doi.org/10.5772/58491
Edited by Öner Özdemir

Contributors

Hosni Salem, Camila Alves, Luiz Antonio Del Ciampo, Miguel Labay Matías, Nick Zavras, Christos Salakos, K. Velaoras, Şenay (Ok) Çetinkaya, Emine Erçin, Sibel Kuşdemir

Published by InTech

Janeza Trdine 9, 51000 Rijeka, Croatia

Publishing Process Manager Iva Simcic

Technical Editor InTech DTP team

Cover InTech Design team

First published February, 2015

Printed in Croatia

Additional hard copies can be obtained from orders@intechopen.com

Pediatric Nursing, Psychiatric and Surgical Issues , Edited by Öner Özdemir

p. cm.

ISBN 978-953-51-1740-7

For EU product safety concerns:
IN TECH d.o.o., Prolaz Marije Krucifikse Kozulić 3, 51000 Rijeka, Croatia,
info@intechopen.com or visit our website at intechopen.com.

Meet the editor

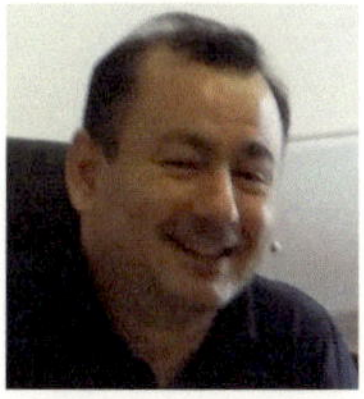

Prof. Dr. Oner Özdemir was born in Alaplı, Zonguldak, Turkey in 1965. He has graduated from İstanbul Medical School, İstanbul University and became a medical doctor in 1989. Dr. Özdemir did his pediatric residency at Department of Pediatrics in Children's Hospital, İstanbul Medical School, İstanbul, Turkey. His clinical fellowship training was completed at Pediatric Allergy/Immunology division in Louisiana State University, Health Sciences Centre, New Orleans, LA. Dr. Özdemir bench research areas are as follows: LAK-cell generation and cell-mediated cytotoxicity; human mast cell development and mast cell-mediated cytotoxicity; and apoptosis related research. He was the first place winner of Clemens Von Pirquet Award from ACAAI at ACAAI meeting in 2005 for the best research on Allergy/Asthma/Immunology by a fellow in training. Dr. Özdemir has more than 60 international and 35 national publications, as well as 100 international and 65 national presentations, and more than 8 chapters related to his research areas. He has been an editor of 4 books so far. Currently, he works as a Head of Pediatrics of the Division of Pediatric Allergy/Immunology at Medical Faculty of Sakarya University, Sakarya Research and Training Hospital, Adapazarı, Sakarya, Turkey.

Contents

Preface

It has been a great honor for me to be an editor of the book titled *'Pediatric Nursing, Psychiatric and Surgical Issues'* , after being editor of "Contemporary Pediatrics" and "Complementary Pediatrics" a couple of years ago.

The book is not a classic pediatric text book. It shows different approaches to some pediatric topics. Our aim in this book, as understood from its title, is to describe some specific issues related to nursing, psychiatric and surgical issues. The book *'Pediatric Nursing, Psychiatric and Surgical Issues'* has 8 chapters which are placed in 4 different sections, to enlighten patients and pediatricians on current developments on specific pediatric issues.

After discussing 'Pediatrics, the People and Politicians in Spain' in our earlier book titled 'Contemporary Pediatrics', here, as the founder of modern pediatrics in Spain, Andrés Martínez Vargas was presented by Dr. Miguel under the section of History of Pediatrics.

Under the second (Nursing Issues) section, Dr. Şenay Çetinkaya tells on nursing approaches for food allergies and osteomyelitis. These two chapters are very interesting to our pediatrician readers since pediatricians are always told and thought about medical care given by physicians. Here, they will learn about nursing approaches in food allergies and osteomyelitis, which are written by a pediatric nursing lecturer.; Prof. Luiz Antonio describes nonintentional injury prevention in children.

Under the third (pediatric psychiatry) section, the psychological problems seen in children of divorced parents, the nursing approach is delineated by Dr. Çetinkaya. Also, Prof. Camila explains chronic health conditions in childhood and adolescence and the formation of care and support networks. These chapters are supportive to the sections of pediatric surgery and psychosocial issues in our earlier book 'Complementary Pediatrics'.

Under the fourth (pediatric surgery) section, Prof. Hosni discusses and tries to solve dilemma in teenager varicocele; Dr. Zavras Nick updates management strategies of short-bowel syndrome in children.

In conclusion, with these 8 chapters, this book enlightens pediatricians on different and less-known issues of pediatric subspecialty one more time.

Before I finish my say here, I am indebted to my mother *Nikâme* , beloved wife *Seval Hülya* and my daughter *Berrin Nikâme* for their precious support during the editing process of time.

Öner Özdemir, MD
Head and Professor of Pediatrics,
Department of Pediatrics, Division of Allergy and Immunology,
Research and Training Hospital of Sakarya University,
Faculty of Medicine, Sakarya University,
Adapazarı, Sakarya, Turkey

Section 1

History of Pediatrics

Chapter 1

Andrés Martínez Vargas, the Founder of Modern Paediatrics in Spain

Miguel Labay Matías

Additional information is available at the end of the chapter

http://dx.doi.org/10.5772/58889

1. Introduction

Unlike the history of Spain, which has been the subject of many studies and publications by authors of recognised prestige, the history of Spanish medicine in general, and of Spanish paediatrics in particular, are not well known to the wider world. The contributions to our scientific heritage made by several Spanish doctors are plentiful, pioneering and important. Andrés Martínez Vargas (1861-1948) is considered the founder of modern Spanish paediatrics. His extensive work is not valued highly enough and he still remains in the shadows. This text is intended to be a fitting tribute to his fascinating life and works.

As a result, the author has carefully read many of his texts, drawing conclusions that aim to show the real nature of this master of paediatrics, one who loved his country.

2. The first stages in his life

Writing about Professor Andrés Martínez Vargas means writing about the founder of modern paediatrics in Spain. His personal life and career present so many facets that it is difficult to summarise them.

He was born in 1861 in the city of Barbastro, in the province of Huesca. Barbastro is for many the main point of entry from the Aragon region to the Central Pyrenees. The oldest of seven children, and the son of a barber in the city, whose establishment was located in the central Plaza del Mercado market square, he clearly stood out in his primary school studies at the Colegio de los Padres Escolapios School in Barbastro. He was first cousin to the acclaimed *regenerationist* and thinker Joaquín Costa Martínez (1846-1911). Joaquín Costa was a great

Spanish visionary, a fighter, an idealist, who coined phrases like "*escuela, despensa y siete llaves para el sepulcro del Cid*" (school, larder and double-lock the tomb of El Cid). With his ideas he was instrumental in the first Spanish irrigation systems, public works, the Europeanisation of Spain and he always felt close to the people he served until his death. Despite the age difference, this man, with whom Andrés Martínez Vargas had a close relationship, must have been a role model for him [1, 2].

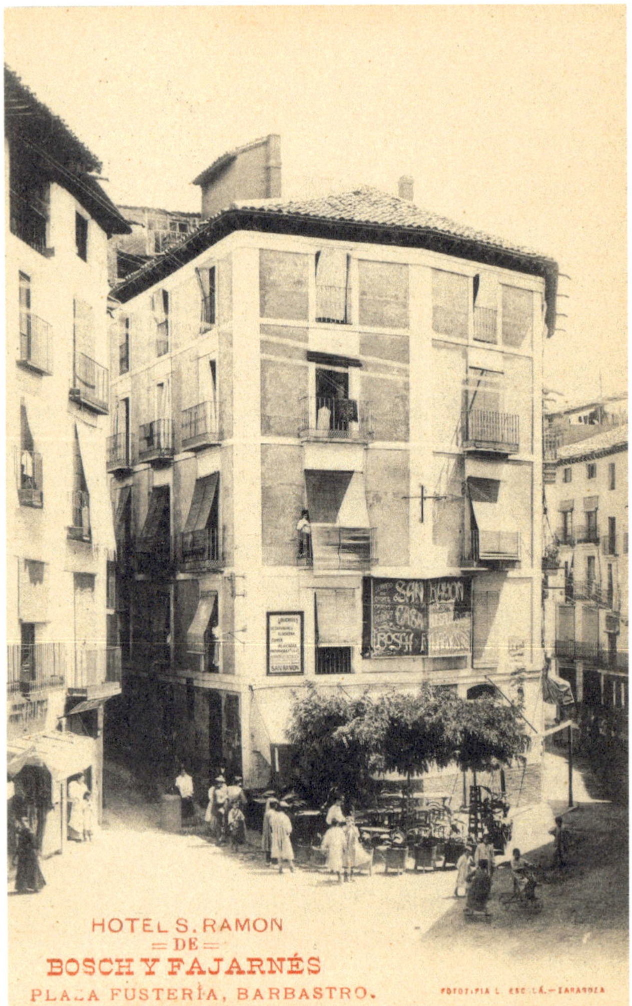

Figure 1. Barbastro (Huesca), at the end of XIX century. El Cruzado Aragonés archives

With no medical background in the family, in 1877 he began studying medicine at the University of Zaragoza, finishing his studies at the age of nineteen with an Outstanding grade and Extraordinary Degree Award. He moved to Madrid and, under the supervision of Doctor José Salamero Martínez, defended his doctoral thesis (1881) "*Clorosis: crítica de sus teorías*

http://dx.doi.org/10.5772/58889

patogénicas" (Chlorosis: review of its pathogenic theories), obtaining the highest possible qualification. His teacher, Doctor Antonio Espina y Capó, suggested that he put himself forward for the public entrance exams to work in the *Cuerpo de Beneficencia* (General Charity Society) in Madrid, and he was offered one of the five jobs available, for which 105 people had applied [3].

3. The beginnings

He was not idle during his time in the Spanish capital. He worked for the Charity, at the University, and with Juan R. Gómez Pano and Antonio Espina y Capó, acting as third signatory in the selection and drafting of articles on medicine, pharmaceuticals and official notices in various volumes of *"La Oficina de Farmacia Española"* (The Spanish Pharmacy). This vast body of work is worth examining to understand the surprising world of healthcare and its pharmacopoeia all around the globe in the late nineteenth century [4]. It is equivalent to thinking about the Internet today. It includes chapters about Healthcare Legislation, all kinds of lists of subjects for public entrance exams, pharmacology, toxicology, hydrotherapy, medicines, new equipment, supply of books, etc. It also had correspondents in all the provinces and many countries, some still Spanish Colonies overseas, as well as in France, England and Germany, and they sent back huge amounts of information for articles. What cannot fail to draw attention is the widespread use of opium, cannabis and cocaine in many preparations. Curing was difficult at that time and instead doctors listened and relieved. I cannot resist reproducing some examples of this. *"Whooping cough, the treatment of: Administer a common or coffee spoonful, according to the child's age, of the following solution in the morning and afternoon in a glass of milk to which an egg yolk has been added: 2 grams of potassium bromide, 4 grams of sodium, 2 grams of ammonia, 6 grams of codeine, 60 grams of water, 50 grams of chloral syrup (Le Nouveau Remédes, 8 February 1886)". "Coryza (the treatment of): 1 gram of cocaine hydrochloride, Water, Glycerine up to 10 grams. Bathe the nasal passages with a cotton bud. The coryza is cured instantly, even in children (Barataux, 1887)." "Cocaine pills: Cocaine hydrochloride 16 parts, powdered opium 64, Menthol 16, Marshmallow root 48. Mix them according to the recipe with glycerine and gum arabic. This is for making pills of 3 centigrams in weight, to be placed on the decayed tooth. Immediate effect in all ages (Zeitschrift d. Allg. Ap. Ver., 1888).* There are chapters like that on saccharin, among others, that are written by Antonio Espina and Andrés Martínez Vargas. The issue I consulted contains more than 1, 500 pages.

4. His time in America

His restless spirit led him to abandon Madrid (1886). He was already particularly interested in illnesses that affect children. Therefore he travelled to the USA, to the Bellevue Hospital, to have classes and practice medicine with the acclaimed Abraham Jacobi, considered the grandfather of American paediatrics. After a two-year stay, he moved to Mexico where he worked and gave talks that allowed him to become part of the Mexican Royal Academy of

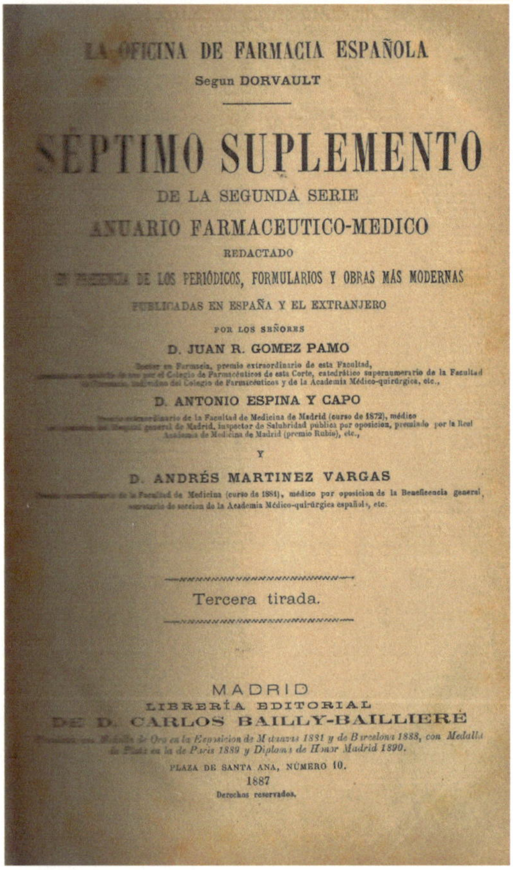
LA OFICINA DE FARMACIA ESPAÑOLA
Segun DORVAULT
SEPTIMO SUPLEMENTO
DE LA SEGUNDA SERIE
ANUARIO FARMACEUTICO-MEDICO
REDACTADO
DE LOS PERIÓDICOS, FORMULARIOS Y OBRAS MÁS MODERNAS
PUBLICADAS EN ESPAÑA Y EL EXTRANJERO
POR LOS SEÑORES
D. JUAN R. GOMEZ PAMO
en Farmacia, premio extraordinario de esta Facultad,
por el Colegio de Farmacéuticos de esta Corte, catedrático supernumerario de la Facultad
del Colegio de Farmacéuticos y de la Academia Médico-quirúrgica, etc.,
D. ANTONIO ESPINA Y CAPO
de la Facultad de Medicina de Madrid (curso de 1872), médico
general de Madrid, inspector de Salubridad pública por oposicion, premiado por la Real
de Medicina de Madrid (premio Rubio), etc.,
Y
D. ANDRÉS MARTINEZ VARGAS
de la Facultad de Medicina (curso de 1881), médico por oposicion de la Beneficencia general,
de seccion de la Academia Médico-quirúrgica española, etc.

Tercera tirada.

MADRID
LIBRERÍA EDITORIAL
DE D. CARLOS BAILLY-BAILLIERE
de Oro en la Exposicion de Matanzas 1881 y de Barcelona 1888, con Medalla
en la de Paris 1889 y Diploma de Honor Madrid 1890.
PLAZA DE SANTA ANA, NÚMERO 10.
1887
Derechos reservados.

Figure 2. The Spanish Pharmacy. Property of author

Medicine. He rejected the good financial deals they offered him and returned to Spain. He described it in the following way: *"I travelled to North America in 1886, then from New York to Veracruz, and in that city and in Mexico I was offered two well-paid medical positions, which I did not accept as I only wanted to serve Spain......."* [5]. Once back in his country, he learned that vacancies for university professors in *Childhood Illnesses* had been announced. In almost no time, he prepared for the public entrance exams and obtained the job at the University of Granada (1888). Only one year earlier, Patricio Borobio, who would become a lifelong friend, had obtained the same position in Zaragoza.

5. University professor in Granada

In Granada he founded the *"School for Mothers"* in order to educate them on how to take better care of their children. He was alarmed by the poverty and the lack of health education common throughout Spain at that time. He had already suggested that the subject he taught should

http://dx.doi.org/10.5772/58889

change its name and become known as *Paediatrics*. He was known for his social concerns, visiting the most deprived areas of the city, such as the caves of *Albaicín*, located close to the impressive *Alhambra*, and he began giving informative talks to its inhabitants about personal and family hygiene. He was behind the creation of the institution that was later known as *"Gota de Leche"* (Milk Drop) (1891). These centres were attended by healthy wet nurses who donated their milk. This was then sterilised, stored in cold conditions and administered in bottles to the newborns and infants who needed it [6]. The current Spanish *"Bancos de leche materna"* (Breast milk banks) are their heirs. However, nobody remembers these doctors from the nineteenth century. They were led by Francisco Vidal y Solares (1890) who founded a centre in Barcelona. Years later (in 1904) Rafael Ulecia y Cardona in Madrid would call this the *"Gota de Leche"* and would then start something similar at their own expense (in Barcelona, Granada, Madrid and gradually widening to the remaining Spanish cities). Andrés Martínez Vargas, aware of the great initiative by Francisco Vidal y Solares, introduced it into his *School for Mothers* in Granada. On 2 October 1888 he began his teaching activity and in that Facility established a subject which had not existed until then. His lessons on diarrhoea, diphtheria and infant assessments, etc. were followed with enthusiasm by his students. He developed and published some perimetric and pedi-barometric charts: *"Tabla pedibarométrica como directora de la lactancia y profiláctica de la mortalidad infantil"* (Pedi-barometric table as a guide to breastfeeding and preventing infant mortality). He gave some lessons on the *"Introduction to Paediatrics"*, reinforcing his idea that the subject should be named in this way [7].

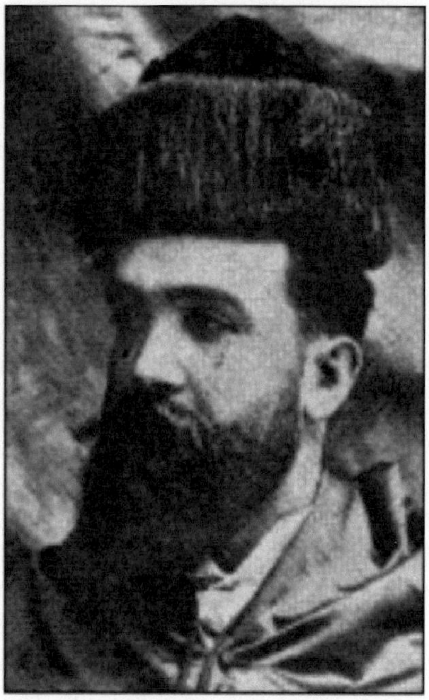

Figure 3. Andrés Martinez Vargas, as young. Property of author

6. University professor in Barcelona

After a rewarding stay, and through a competitive transfer process, he obtained the *Chair of Childhood Illnesses and their Clinic Practice* at the University of Barcelona (1892).

He would live in Barcelona until his death (1948). His activity was extraordinary throughout his professional life. He did not like what he found at the Faculty of Medicine and its Hospital: clutter, filth, lack of medical equipment, lack of space, etc. Everything he achieved was through hard work [8]. He joined the *Real Academia de Medicina de Cataluña* (Royal Academy of Medicine of Catalonia) in 1894 with the talk "*Empyema in children*", actively participating in its sessions.

7. Initiative to create a ministry of health

One of his most famous speeches was given at the Commemorative Session of the 150th Anniversary of the Royal Academy of Medicine, held on 29 December 1920.

This speech was entitled "*The Ministry of Health in Spain*" [9]. He began his speech by noting that this Academic Corporation was older than the ones in London and Paris. He argued brilliantly: *"Social medicine is the combination of medical knowledge and the legislative progress, directly applied to the welfare of the individual and social improvement. Ideally its purpose is to reduce disease and mortality, prolong average life expectancy, especially in the lower classes....My view is that the new age will be characterised by greater interest in the physical and mental health of man and by the direct involvement of medicine in the governing of towns.... Given all of this, it can be argued that in times of peace as in those of war, the health of the citizens is the most important factor in work, wealth and progress... all the gold on earth would not be enough to restore life to a dead person...man spends half his life mining the natural resources of his health, and the other half making desperate efforts to recover the good that has been lost"*. He was upset that in Spain infant mortality in children under one year of age was 157 deaths per 1, 000 in 1917 (twice that of Holland, Denmark, Norway, etc.) and that up to five years it stood at 45 percent. He railed against the mass emigration of Spaniards (56, 400 in the first half of 1920) along with the alarming birth rate, the low population density, the indiscriminate abortions, the filthiness of grocery stores, the poor sanitation of housing, its high prices, the total lack of control over drinking water, the lack of interest from politicians in improving the situation by legislating and enforcing laws....He ended by saying: *"If order and plans are the essential basis for success, and dissociation that for failure, there is no doubt that Spain, with the current fragmented system of medical responsibilities, cannot improve on what already exists. The secular organisation of healthcare reveals an infinite dispersion of factors that involve the Ministries of Interior, War, Justice, Development, Education, and others....This dispersion of power and responsibility brings with it a loss of energy, inefficiency, irresponsibility, mutual excuses for mistakes, disorientation in censoring and the impossibility of remedies... to which we can add the little interest shown by Deputies and Senators in the issue... This is why we need to create the Ministry of Health in Spain, following the examples of France and England. This request had already been made in 1910, at the First International Congress on tuberculosis in Barcelona..."*. The criticism of politicians was bitter and blunt: *"A former Minister of the Crown has denounced once again the contempt and disdain with which many Ministers and MPs have treated health issues, and has highlighted the supine ignorance that places them at the level of a bad Medical student. When it comes to health problems they behave badly due to a lack of understanding of the problem… The leaders of the country are more interested in other businesses that are more lucrative to them...but we must not lose hope... I believe Spain should be part of the Red Cross with all its consequences".* Andrés, a great visionary, anticipated by more than 70 years the creation of the Ministry of Health in Spain. Some of his phrases and arguments are still valid today.

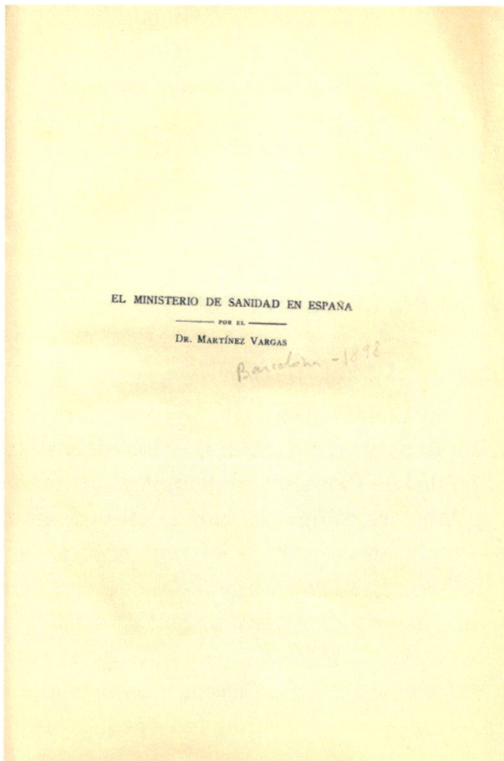

EL MINISTERIO DE SANIDAD EN ESPAÑA

POR EL

DR. MARTÍNEZ VARGAS

Figure 4. Ministerio de Sanidad: Discourse. Property of author

8. His journal and social concerns

We now go back to 1900 when he founded the scientific journal *"La Medicina de los niños"* (Medicine for children), in which he, along with other authors, published countless articles until 1936. Many of them are cited by the author in numerous published books and talks. The Spanish civil war put an end to this scientific journal, as it did to all of them [2, 7].

He spoke French, English and German and had a good grasp of Russian. This allowed him to be the main Spanish scientific ambassador in many conferences and meetings of all kinds.

There is a record of more than 300 articles published and signed by Andrés, many of them in English, French and German. He collaborated with "La Vanguardia" (Barcelona) and other newspapers, producing another 500 informative articles on aspects of hygiene, disease prevention, child care and care for mothers. Some of them can still be found on the Internet [2].

Deeply concerned about the lack of health and general culture in the majority of the population, he organised and played a leading role in *"La Universidad Popular"* (The People's University-1902), where on Sunday mornings he would offer free informative talks to the most disadvantaged people in Barcelona's industrial belt. His obsession was to improve the level of education. Other notable scientists such as Odón de Buen from Zaragoza also took part. Not content with this initiative, he imported the idea of the German *"Kindergarten"*, so that working mothers would have places where their young children could be looked after and breastfed by their mothers. In short, he was the promoter of the first Spanish nurseries. At the same time he fought for working women to be given enough time to breastfeed their children and for them to be fed [1, 2, 6, 7, 10].

9. His relationship with doctor Julio Comby

In 1896, he translated the Treatise on *"Enfermedades de la Infancia"* (Childhood Illnesses) by the famous French physician Julio Comby [11]. The copy I have read belonged to Dr Alfredo Cebrián. The quality and depth of what is written is of the highest level for its time. Interestingly, Andrés added and published footnotes containing many extremely valuable personal observations, notes and explanatory comments, along with contributions from other foreign authors. Dr Comby wrote about breastfeeding: *"Natural breastfeeding should be continued for sixteen to eighteen months, while there is no problem for the mother, since there can be none for the child during this time; on the contrary, the longer breastfeeding continues, the stronger the child will become. It shall be exclusive in the first eight or ten months; only from that age may the child be given some easily digestible foods, such as rice flour, tapioca.... They must not be given wine, vinous water or coffee; milk must be their ordinary beverage, not only during breastfeeding but also long after weaning..."*. Doctor Cebrián wrote a footnote in pencil: *"Dr Martínez Vargas thought the same in his recent speech at the Ateneo" [11].*

In the chapter on diphtheria, the historical quotations from Andrés highlight the ignorance that existed about Spanish medical history on this and other topics. *"As the author has outlined, in terms of the history of diphtheria, Spanish literature has been very fruitful on this matter and I feel it necessary to record here my personal research that I shared at the 12th International Medical Congress held in Moscow in August 1897. The result of that work has been the rehabilitation of Spanish physicians from the sixteenth and seventeenth centuries, both before the assembly and in the medical literature due to the fact that the main conclusions of my paper are recorded in the recent work by the Professor of Paediatrics in Berlin, A. Bagynsky: Diphterie und Diphteristicher croup, Vienna 1898, on page 4... Despite Spain being the country where the clinical description of diphtheria took place, almost all historians omit the work of Spanish physicians on this and other diseases... The first description of croup also came from Spanish authors in the first*

http://dx.doi.org/10.5772/58889

third of the sixteenth century, using the name "garrotillo" or "morbo sofocante" (gallows disease). What follows is a historical journey which quotes, in detail, Pedro Díaz de Toledo, Luis Lobera de Ávila, Jerónimo Soriano (for his masterful description of tonsillitis), Luis de Mercado, Francisco Vallés, Cristóbal Pérez Herrera, Juan de Soto, Francisco Pérez Cascales, Juan Alonso de los Ruices y Fontecha, Alfonso Nuñez, Francisco Figueroa and Antonio Pérez de Escobar. The text covers five pages. He also provides his personal experience with cases of recurrent diphtheria. He fought the idea that an attack of diphtheria provides protection for life. He advocated the administration of an anti-diphtheria serum and suggested that children's immune systems required repeated administrations of the serum to prevent very serious episodes which could kill them [11].

With regards to measles, Dr Comby says: *"In this case I have a very eloquent example that reinforces much of the author's advice. I refer to a three-year old girl who, due to being neglected by her relatives in the first twelve hours of the eruptive period of measles, had difficulty with the outbreak of the spots; very soon her temperature rose to 41° and 42°, and then she suffered violent eclamptic fits, with asystole and very intense cyanosis; given the imminence of death I decided to give cold affusions with iced water for half an hour; the fever broke, and this very complex clinical incident calmed down, the disease could once again run its course and the eruption broke out, splendidly, all across the skin's surface; the girl was cured in the same way as with regular forms of the disease".*

When writing about childhood tuberculosis, Dr Comby concluded that its prognosis is one of the bleakest as it may lie dormant until it manifests itself in adolescence or adulthood. It was already known that Koch's bacillus was the cause of this terrible pandemic. The author of the Treatise wrote: "... *When the liver and spleen are of a considerable volume, especially if the spleen comes through the false ribs and is clearly visible in the abdomen, you can almost confirm the presence of tuberculosis"*. Andrés, added: *"In certain cases the examination of temperature can be of great service. After numerous observations I could convince myself that in latent tuberculosis there is a temperature under 37° for long periods; and this prolonged hypothermia, combined with other symptoms, will serve to reveal the existence of hidden tuberculosis....This hypothermia is persistent. I have discovered twelve cases in children and young people with these characteristics, which were confirmed later (De l'hipothermie dans la tuberculose, sa valeur diagnostique. Congrès de Obstetrique et de Pediatrie-Burdeos, August, 1895, page. 1005).*

Martínez Vargas claimed that the diagnosis of tuberculous meningitis was very simple. Martínez Vargas advised that after carrying out the lumbar puncture, the cerebral spinal fluid should be placed in a test tube and kept for one or two days at room temperature. At the end of this time, a *"little cloud"* appeared at the top of the liquid. He stated that in this *"little cloud"* it is very easy to observe microscopic Koch's bacilli. This "little cloud" is a fibrin network in which the bacilli are concentrated, and these can be identified quickly and safely. He may not have been the discoverer, but he spread the word in Spain. This method has been used by the signatory in the cases of tuberculous meningitis attended and it has never failed. The problem of how to rapidly diagnose tuberculous meningitis was solved more than one hundred years ago, but has been lost to current generations. It would be a wise move to recover it [12].

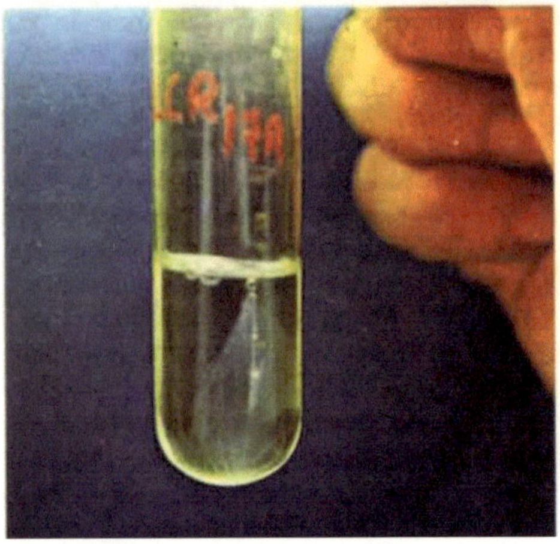

Figure 5. Fibrin network. Source: http://www.actamedicacolombiana.com/anexo/articulos/01-1976-05.htm

The description of onanism by Doctor Comby is very curious, as he says it is a disturbance in genital feeling that is observed in both sexes even at very early ages, without deserving the importance given to it in general. He explains that in girls it may be caused by pruritus vulvae or the presence of pinworms. Although he describes the morbid consequences of the act: *"emaciation, paleness, ineptitude in all physical and intellectual efforts... however we should not take against the onanists... it is better to offer them a healthy lifestyle, with exercise and outdoor games... the nervous and agitated will be given potassium bromide. In girls female circumcision has been proposed and practised, successfully"!!!...* Andrés makes no comment, which is significant and could be considered as an expression of his disapproval.

In today's culture, the previous paragraph by the French physician would be unacceptable. Nonetheless, the Treatise is full of wisdom. The chapter dealing with Kidney Diseases is fantastic for its content. In the chapter devoted to Bladder stones, our protagonist added: *"... in one of the operations that I performed on a child in the clinic in Granada in the year 1889, I found a stone very attached to the mucous, not encapsulated, and this character, not mentioned before that time, should form an integral part of this pathological chapter. To learn all about this process, see my work,* **Adherent vesical calculus in a child**, *published with engravings in The Archives of Pediatrics, Philadelphia, April 1890".* This article was the first in Spanish history to be published by a paediatrician in an American journal. Later there would be others published in English, French and German. [11] It was quoted in the fourth edition of the Treatise of Paediatrics by the German Doctor Luis Unger. However, it was not mentioned in previous editions [13].

10. Interest in basic school education

In 1905, he published his *"Botiquín Escolar"* (School First-Aid Kit), in the *La Escuela Moderna* (The Modern School) publications. It was a small manual which outlined the most common

http://dx.doi.org/10.5772/58889

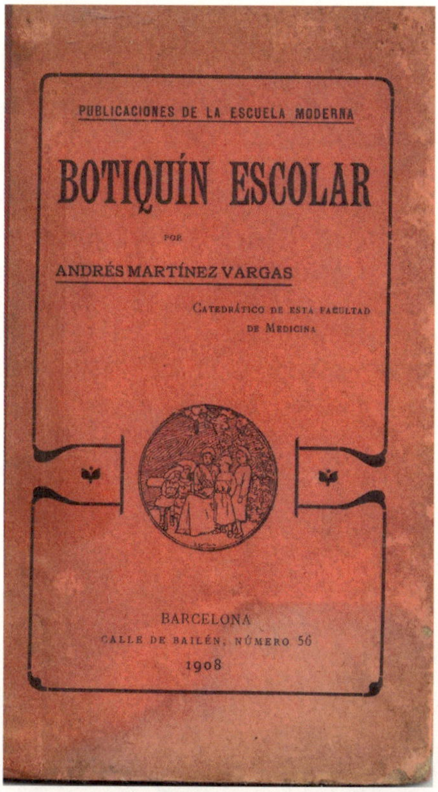

Figure 6. School First-Aid Kit. Property of author

problems faced by children during their time at school [14]. It has 14 chapters and consists of everything required to provide assistance to pupils as and when needed. It was priced at 0.50 peseta centimos. For the first time the manoeuvres for basic cardiopulmonary resuscitation were explained, through text and drawings, and it advised that children who have suffered a blow to the head, suffering from mild concussion, should be allowed to sleep, against popular belief, and said that placing a coin pressed against the "bump" was not appropriate. It is written with a lot of common sense. *"Understanding how to prevent children having accidents and how to cure the sudden ailments they may suffer in their daily school life is of such importance that teachers have made it known to me...I have been unable to explain the omission of those writing about Hygiene in schools with regards to the Boletín Escolar (School Newsletter). Neither in theory has their involvement been advised, nor in practice has there been any teaching about this issue. However, in few places is the helpfulness of having at hand a number of resources which serve to remedy the various accidents that children may experience whilst at school been so evident. As a result of the Hygiene talks that I have been giving at the Escuela Moderna (Modern School) for four years now, I have become convinced of how regrettable this omission is, and therefore, that the First-aid kit is as necessary as any other school item… It seems to me that this First-aid kit should be found in every teaching institution, whatever its nature, and that teachers and senior students should be familiarised with its handling... so that nobody can say due to ignorance or neglect: that the remedy is one hundred times worse than the disease".*

11. Interesting personal details

There are certain endearing aspects about the life of Andrés. During his time as a medical student in Zaragoza, he stayed in lodgings in the street called *calle Prudencio,* owned by my great grandmother. In the nineteen eighties demolition men destroyed the entire area. Later, once working as a university professor, he was a regular customer of the El Sol Hotel on his visits to the capital located on the Ebro River. The Hotel, run by my grandparents, was in the street *calle Alfonso,* on the corner with the street *calle Molino,* very close to the Basilica of Nuestra Señora del Pilar (Our Lady of the Pillar). This building still exists today, now converted into apartments. My grandparents told me that Andrés was a polite and charming man, with a very healthy appetite. The daily menu consisted of five courses and he loved to have second helpings. Later he would stay at the Gran Hotel, but frequently returned to visit this old hotel [1, 2]. His great-grandson, Andrés Martínez-Vargas Vallés, told me that when he was older he would eat an entire chicken on Sundays. When reprimanded by his wife, Ángeles Mariana, he would exclaim: "Woman, it is mostly bones".

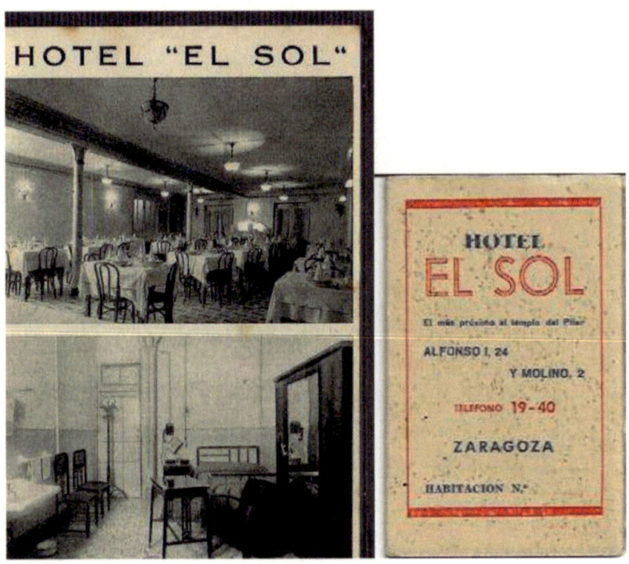

Figure 7. El Sol Hotel and accommodation card. Property of author

12. Typhoid fever

Of great interest is "*Tratamiento de la Fiebre tifoidea con el Suero. Publicaciones de la Medicina de los Niños*" (Treatment of Typhoid fever with Serum. Publications from Medicine for Children) (1910). The copy I have read is personally dedicated by the author to the prestigious General Valeriano Weyler [15]. It describes fourteen cases, with great accuracy, in a clinical lecture given on 11 December 1909, with bibliographic notes on articles published in various languages. Its prologue reads as follows: *"In this booklet I explain my clinical studies on curing typhoid fever using an anti-typhoid serum and demonstrate the undisputed usefulness of the anti-typhoid vaccine. The curing of typhoid fever with the serum is a fact. This terrible disease, painful due to its duration, repugnance, complications, irremediable injuries and high mortality, can be cured with a simple injection of the serum, a relatively benign treatment...I seek satisfaction for my country with Spain having been the first nation in the world in whose medical press these anti-typhoid serum studies have appeared. The publication of two articles of mine in La Gaceta médica Catalana and in la Medicina de los Niños (1909) have been the first that I know of, published in the press in Spain and abroad... Typhoid fever has produced more casualties than steel, lead and shrapnel... Having demonstrated its transmission by water and inter-human infection, and that convalescents can spread infectious bacilli through their faeces or urine 2 and 3 weeks after being cured…The vaccination of health staff is required, in nursing homes, in families...Serum for the sick and vaccinations for the healthy."* With this our protagonist demonstrates his scientific greatness and his national pride.

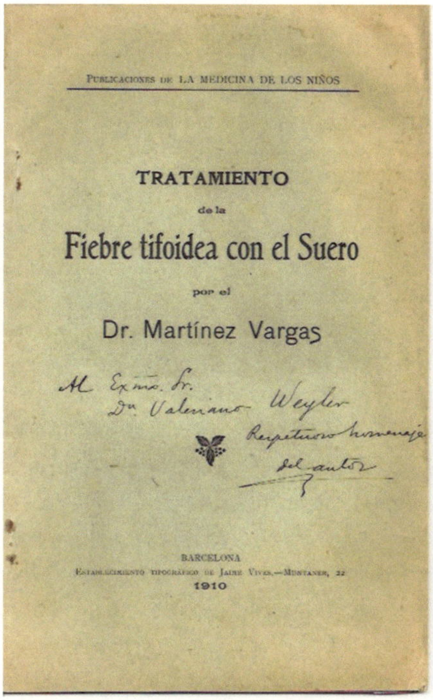

Figure 8. Treatment of Typhoid fever with Serum. Publications from Medicine for Children. Property of author

13. Criticism of the Spanish situation at that time and his proposals

In 1918 he gave the Inaugural Address at the solemn opening of the Academic Year before the Faculty at the University of Barcelona. Its title *"In defence of race"*, may be viewed as controversial in the eyes of modern readers. However, its content is extraordinary and shows the protagonist's social concerns [16]. Once again his personality can be seen from the reasoning and the energy that shines through. *"The older I am, the more I feel the obligation for every citizen to yield to their country and society all the fruit of their experience and their worth, as cooperation in creating the national heritage and as a fair return for the culture with which the nation supported their youth, educated them and prepared them for social action…To my homeland I offer my musings, my work, and some procedures that, if put into practice with great perseverance, will be able to improve our children, our men and put the Spanish nation on a level with the most cultured nations"*

Andrés demonstrated his pure love for Spain, an aspect that a part of the Catalan nationalist bourgeoisie did not accept. However, many of the social, human and scientific initiatives were of particular benefit to Catalonia. After reading many of his texts, I have come to the conclusion that he was a person of deep religious belief, who had a conservative nature but very advanced social ideas for his time. This dichotomy makes him an even more interesting figure. His pioneering initiatives in human affairs, his boundless dedication to the most disadvantaged, defending the rights of women and children, and of the workers, are examples of this. He did not like what he saw and experienced in Spain, so he fought against it to improve its position. He was conservative in some ways, but extremely progressive in everything social. Multilingual, with people skills, intelligence, a lucid mind that accepted and adopted ideas, a way with words and a gifted writer, researcher, innovator, tireless worker, risk taker, a brave man, interested in everything and everyone, with his own ideas, dedicated to children, families and his beloved Spain and Catalonia, which he fought to improve: that was Andrés.

He continues: *"Over recent centuries Spanish society has ignored the regressive reality, living in a continuous paradox with a superficial appearance of strength that concealed a weak interior, with no resistance or austerity; we thought we were invincible until this was tested...but the summer of 1898 came and the country emerged from its historical party to face a surprise: with the disaster the nation lost over half its territory and all its legendary prestige. Since that moment all lips, all speeches, and all printed pages have been full of cries of great pain and an intense national crisis with a strong yearning for improvement has been revealed. Our rulers, the ones who must fix this problem, have sharpened their wits devising a more or less sonorous phrase as a remedy for everything, with no decisive action; one after another they have limited themselves to squeezing the lexicon to create new words that by dint of repetition have fallen into vulgarity and blandness... and with this policy of phrases twenty years have passed aggravating the problem…"*. These phrases, pronounced in 1918, have also not lost their validity when looking at the situation today. He summarised the Spanish situation at that time: famine, basic lack of culture, lack of hygiene, little importance placed on a child's life, growth deficiency in the Spanish in comparison with the Europeans, the terrifying infant mortality figures already explained previously, multiple authorities that make the country ungovernable.... He wrote something that is very curious but true: *"We physicians who help children know the great value of the relationship between an observant mother and the manifestations of a disease in their children, as on many occasions they have given us half the diagnosis"*.

http://dx.doi.org/10.5772/58889

He strongly argued that the basis of the recovery of Spain was in schools, food and healthcare [16]. He listed the needs of children and adolescents according to age. He proposed the creation of an "Ethnocultural Commission", along the lines of the local and provincial boards of education. He spoke of his *Child Protection Policies*, established in Lleida, through which parents signed a commitment to do their utmost to keep their children alive until they reached the age of one, for which they were financially rewarded. "*We must put an end to the laws appearing in La Gaceta and not regulating our actions... no child should leave school until they are at least 12 years old. If they show their skills they should be rewarded with State or private scholarships… a country that wastes more than 2, 000, 000 pesetas in horse racing and quadruple that in bullfighting should not find it difficult to organise a loan of 30, 000, 000 for schools and scholarships...the prosperity of a people depends more on its education system than on its institutions or government. To fulfil this duty, there is no need for new laws, new agencies, newly appointed civil servants, or financial sacrifices: the will to achieve it and to organise the resources already there is enough.*" One would think that he was writing about modern-day Spain. Due to extension problems it is impossible to say what he thinks about teachers. One hundred years ago he was already arguing for what is currently required: vocation, knowledge, ability to teach, observing the behaviour of children even in the playground, treating them according to their characteristics, and he concludes by saying that these are the basis of the educational system. This speech is so rich in concepts and development that it deserves a chapter of its own [16].

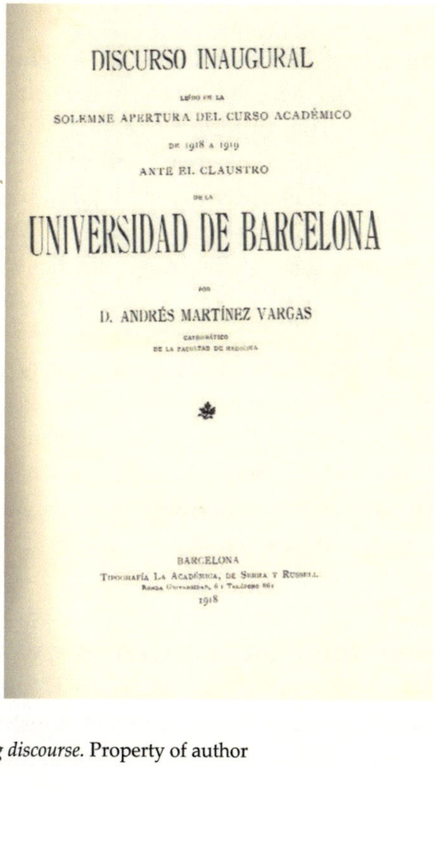
DISCURSO INAUGURAL

SOLEMNE APERTURA DEL CURSO ACADÉMICO

ANTE EL CLAUSTRO

UNIVERSIDAD DE BARCELONA

D. ANDRÉS MARTÍNEZ VARGAS

BARCELONA

1918

Figure 9. *In defence of race: Opening discourse.* Property of author

14. Various initiatives and awards

He founded the Catalonia Society of Paediatrics and the Spanish Society of Paediatrics (1912) which, although it had a short life, is the origin of the current Spanish Association of Paediatrics. He organised and chaired the First National Congress of Paediatrics (Palma de Mallorca 1914). He wrote his impressive *Tratado de Pediatría* (Treatise of Paediatrics) in 1915. He founded the *Instituto Nipiológico* (Nipiological Institute) in Barbastro (1916), which spread throughout the whole of Spain. He was Dean of the Faculty of Medicine and Rector of the University of Barcelona (1921-1927), publicly criticising the lack of interest among students and the neglect of some teachers [17]. He was Senator-elect for Huesca (1922), Honourable Academician of the Royal Hispanic American Academy of Sciences and Arts (1925), and Knight of the Legion of Honour in France (1926). With the protection of the French Consulate he moved to Pamplona during the disastrous Spanish civil war, working as a physician and Head of the Surgical Ward, innovating in the treatment of "trench foot-Teruel feet" or dry gangrene (1937-1939). In 1941 he published the book *Enfermedades del recién nacido* (Diseases in the newborn), considered the pillar of Spanish Neonatology, and in 1947 he made his last great contribution: *Historia de la Pediatría en España (History of Paediatrics in Spain).* He worked up until the last day of his long life (87 years old).

15. In France during the great war

His curiosity about everything and everyone took him to France during the First Great European War (1914-1918) and it was there that he wrote the book *"Mi visita al frente Francés" (My visit to the French front)* (1919). The copy I have seen is dedicated to a French friend. It strikes me that, despite being dedicated in his own handwriting and with a business card, I had to unstick its pages with a scalpel in order to read it [18]. In short, the friend never read this book in which he describes very innovative surgical techniques in the treatment of the terrible wounds caused by "mustard gas", shells, burns, etc. His thoughts are full of wisdom. *"Humanity will not fully enjoy its welfare whilst peace between the nations is not guaranteed, whilst no restrictions are placed on the excesses of a dictator, whilst a kind of patriarchy for universal balance is not created, so that when someone ambitious, unruly or crazy wants to disturb it, the whole weight of the rest of the world is thrown at them, to make them back down, willingly or by force. Instead of performing evil, through science, it would be better to live in a state of backwardness, in primitive ignorance. Progress and civilisation must be based on respect for the law and the concept of justice. Brute force must not dominate reason…"* As is clear from his words, Andrés was a staunch pacifist and unfortunately these words are still valid today.

16. His love for Spain and fundamental scientific works

He had good people skills which allowed him to form relationships with his fellow medics worldwide. He was outraged to find that the history of Spanish medicine counted for nothing

http://dx.doi.org/10.5772/58889

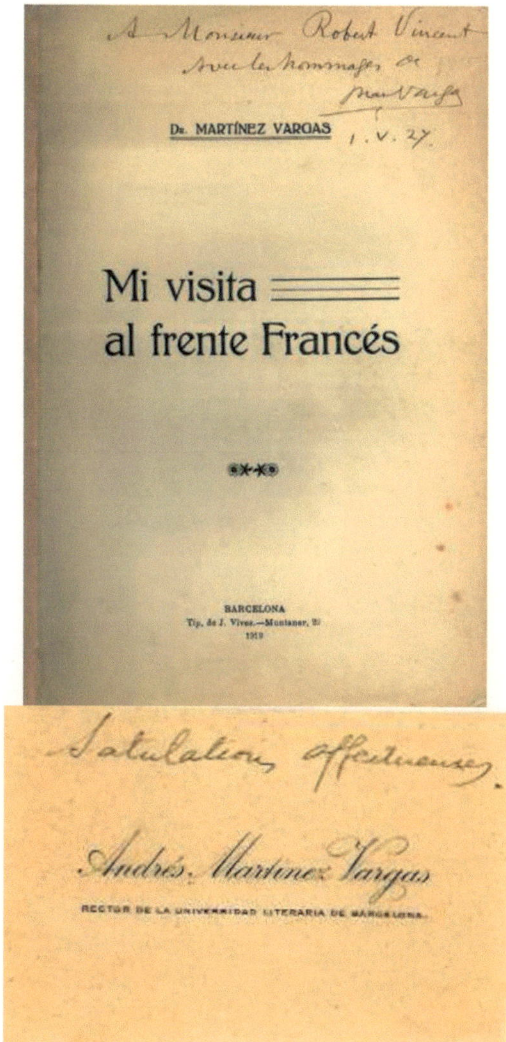

Figure 10. *My visit to the French front* and business card. Property of author

and was systematically ignored. From this blessed indignation arose articles in various prestigious journals, rightly proclaiming the achievements of our medical science. That is the context in which his reflections on the work of the Teruel-born Jerónimo Soriano appeared; they were written in French for a select journal and were not wasted. In the year 1600, his Treatise on Paediatrics, M*ethodo y orden de curar las enfermedades de los niños* (Method and order in curing diseases in children) was published, and Andrés proclaimed him as the very first Spanish and international paediatrician: *"I am going to introduce you to a physician from Aragon, not because I want to endorse regionalism but because he was one of the first doctors in Spain and the world to have written books exclusively about childhood diseases. I am talking about Jerónimo Soriano, born in Teruel, in the final third of the sixteenth century. Soriano belongs to that brilliant age which* *must be considered as the seed for these studies and which constitutes the beginning and foundation of this speciality in Spain and in the whole world".* Andrés heralded the man from Aragon and claimed the rightful place that belonged to his illustrious Spanish physician ancestors, unfairly forgotten inside and outside of Spain. The two greatest founders of Spanish paediatrics had been found…350 years later! [1, 2, 19].

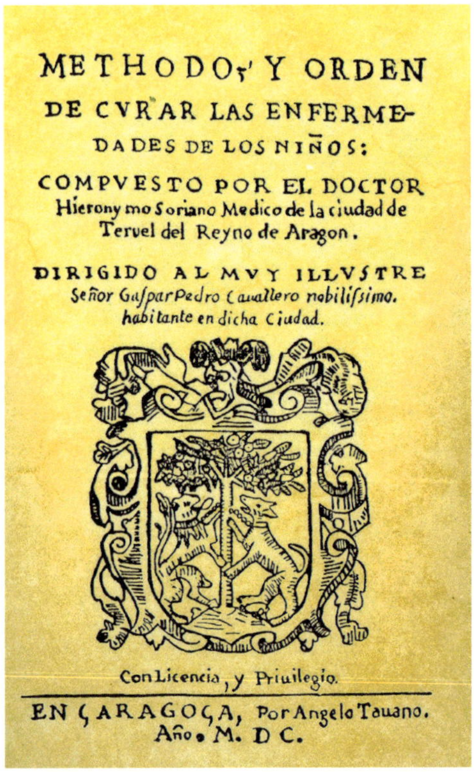
METHODO, Y ORDEN
DE CVRAR LAS ENFERME-
DADES DE LOS NIÑOS:
COMPVESTO POR EL DOCTOR
Hieronymo Soriano Medico de la ciudad de
Teruel del Reyno de Aragon.
DIRIGIDO AL MVY ILLVSTRE
Señor Gaspar Pedro Cauallero nobilissimo.
habitante en dicha Ciudad.
Con Licencia, y Priuilegio.
EN ÇARAGOÇA, Por Angelo Tauano.
Año. M. DC.

Figure 11. Method and order in curing diseases in children, Jerónimo Soriano. Property of author

His major works are the *"Tratado de Pediatría"* (Treatise of Paediatrics) (1915) which he dedicated to his wife and children (*To my beloved wife Angeles Mariana and my children Sara and Andrés)* and *the "Historia de la Pediatría en España"* (History of Paediatrics in Spain) *(1947),* his last major contribution, cited above [8, 17]. In the Prologue of the Treatise, Dr Rodríguez Méndez wrote, among other things: *"I know Martínez Vargas like I know few, or perhaps no, others. With a noble soul, brave spirit, great intelligence, an uncommon culture… Sick or healthy, overwhelmed by his large clientele, he was always the same: a persistent, tireless worker at the forefront of the scientific world...This great student from Aragon made his name in Madrid, in Mexico, in New York...Almost everyone who goes to exotic lands go as an apprentice, only a few return as masters, it is a rare case; Martínez Vargas returned to Spain famous for being a great scholar, a great teacher. They did not teach him abroad: they taught us about his worth. Here he was baptised, but there he was confirmed. He has not rested in the enormous task of championing Paediatrics. I dare to say that his Treatise is the best in existence...*" Reading the Treatise is extremely interesting. Andrés is humble, claiming that you can only take on these tasks with maturity and experience. He defends teaching on three levels: theory, practice and the personal monitoring of the children from the Dispensary in their homes by the students.

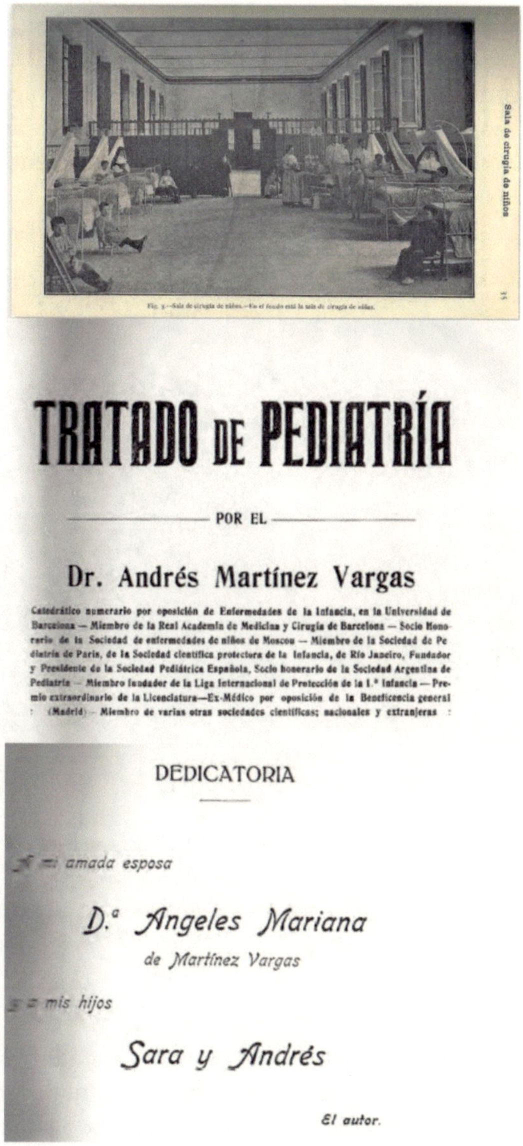

Figure 12. Paediatrics hall, treatise and dedication. Property of author

It is moving to read his informative booklet "*La salud del niño. Consejos a las madres para la mejor crianza de sus hijos*" (A child's health. Advice for mothers to raise their children better). I imagine that at the end of his professional life, in 1946, he wanted to leave a simple and practical legacy for all Spanish families. He writes: *"Every mother has the duty to breastfeed her child. Every child has the right to its mother's breast. When a mother is unable to breastfeed her child, she may be replaced by a wet nurse. If the wet nurse abandons her own child to breastfeed another, she commits an offence against motherhood... A life for a life, no innocent child should be sacrificed!"*. His sensitivity and humanity remain on the record for all time [20]. The table included on the duration of sleep, play and intellectual work for children according to age is very curious. At the age of 7 he recommends one hour of teaching and this increases annually until it reaches eight hours at the age of 14. This makes one think about the children who at early ages are wrongly labelled as being "hyperactive", and "lacking attention", and who over the years adapt to schooling. One might take note, instilling this wisdom in legislators, parents, teachers, professors, psychologists and doctors.

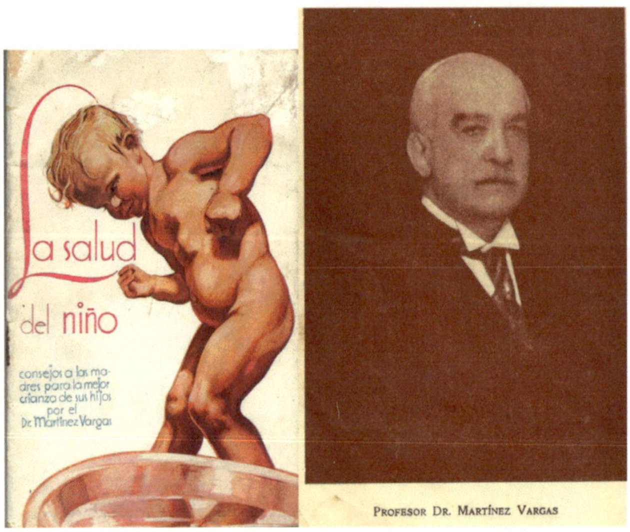

Figure 13. La salud del niño and Andrés Martínez Vargas retired. Property of author

17. Nipiological institute

I was especially impressed by the description of the "*Instituto Nipiológico*" (Nipiological Institute) in Barbastro (1916). The name comes from the word "nipios" in Greek, which means "the one who knows nothing, " referring to the early stages of a child's life. Its founder was the Italian professor, Ernesto Cacace, in 1905. The basis of this doctrine is the need to educate parents on the basic aspects of child care, education, health and nutrition. I do not have the slightest doubt that the choice of Barbastro to found it was an offering to his beloved home town, one full of generosity. *"On 8 September 1918, the city of Barbastro (Huesca) held the third Children's Day. Established in September 1916, it was the first organised in Spain. Infant mortality has decreased by half since its founding. It has involved thirty mothers awarded amounts of 50 pesetas, 40, 30, 20, 15 and less, according to their child's development and how often they attended the Institute; I saw it clearly when creating the Child Protection Policies in 1906 and experience has taught me that prize money is a very effective incentive in attracting mothers to these teaching and assistance establishments; but what I have most effectively seen in these two years at the Institute of Barbastro... The young men of the San Hipólito neighbourhood have even gone without some parties and have donated their money to help the children at this Institute and other charities. Praise be to this Institute which, in addition to protecting children, leads adolescents down the paths of moral perfection!..."* This "invention", imported into Spain by Andrés, was publicised and copied in various Spanish and foreign locations [1, 7, 10].

Professor Cacace from Naples, founder of *Nipiology,* dedicated these words to him at the 3rd Spanish Congress of Paediatrics (Zaragoza, 1925): *"Andrés Martínez Vargas, the grand master of Paediatrics, the supreme apostle of Nipiology, is the leading Spanish figure in this speciality"*. Quite rightly, he described him as the *"Grandfather of Spanish paediatricians and master of them all"*

Another work mentioned previously is "*Enfermedades del niño Recién Nacido*" (Diseases in the newborn child) (1941), one of the first books written specifically about the subject and considered the foundation of Spanish Neonatology.

18. Prologues in various books

He wrote the prologue for many books on different subjects. In "*La voz humana*" (The human voice), he wrote about the need for children and young people to be taught to correctly use their voices, to avoid undesirable consequences, aspects that were personally dealt with in a Course at the Faculty of Medicine. He therefore anticipated Speech Therapy. His love of music in general, and opera in particular, made him talk about three tenors who were leading stars in the nineteenth century: Enrico Tamberlick, the favourite of Queen Isabel II of Spain, Julián Gayarre and Antonio Aramburo [21]. The latter had his voice preserved in the wax cylinders of the time, once retired from the stage. However, he showed his preference for his countryman Miguel Fleta, an exceptional tenor who lived a very short life (he died at 39), but who has bequeathed various examples of unrivalled art for posterity. In another prologue [5], he congratulated the author's father, a pharmacist, for his bravery in defending the freedom of citizens to choose their pharmacy and for having founded, along with his son, some laboratories that were prestigious in their day and which freed Spain from its pharmaceutical dependence on other countries. One anecdote about his interest in music is the event involving the famous Italian tenor Mario del Mónaco in his début at the Gran Teatro del Liceo in Barcelona. Del Mónaco, very young at that time, did not convince his audience who started "hissing" him. Andrés, now elderly, went backstage to greet him, encouraged him and predicted a career full of triumphs due to his powerful and exceptional voice [1]. He told him that at his age he knew a lot about these situations of apparent failure and that he was sure it would serve to drive the tenor on. He was right, and Mario del Mónaco became one of the best dramatic tenors in the history of opera. His revenge was to not return to that stage for a decade. When he did return it was only as a result of a spectacular financial offer.

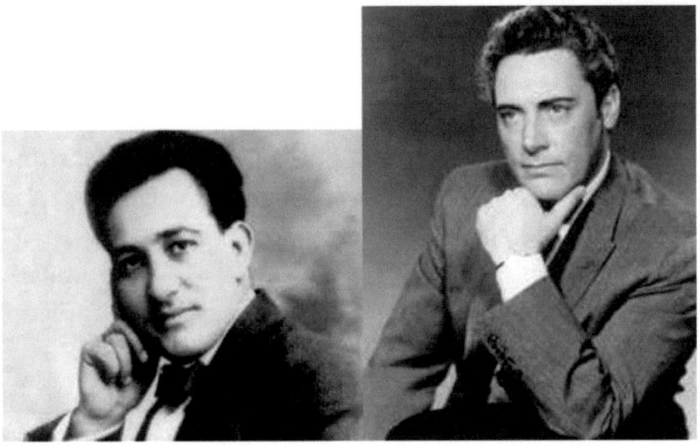

Figure 14. Miguel Fleta and Mario del Mónaco, tenors. Property of author

The impression one gets when looking at the work of Andrés is of his interest and curiosity about medicine, art, humanism, and sociology, his love for children and his desire to serve Spain, his wish to not only improve health care levels but also help society as a whole advance [22].

19. The 1st spanish congress of paediatrics

The 1st Spanish Congress of Paediatrics, held in April 1914 in Palma de Mallorca as a result of his initiative and under his guidance, was a success in terms of many of his professional concerns. It was attended by more than 300 specialists from around the world [7, 23-25]. With this Congress, Paediatrics was consolidated as a speciality. It dealt with various issues relating to Childcare, such as "Insufficient lactic secretion", "Treatment of the umbilical cord", "Breastfeeding and Milk Drops", "The mother's code", the latter being addressed by our protagonist. Issues relating to medicine were also addressed with, among others, the following papers: "Childhood tuberculosis", "Vaccinations", "Dyspepsia" and "Leishmaniosis". Issues relating to Child Surgery were discussed, highlights including the areas of "Scoliosis", "Congenital dislocation of the hip", "Congenital muscular torticollis", "Spina bifida", "Otitis", "Burns" and "Femur fracture". The issue of school hygiene figured prominently in the congressional sessions. Aspects relating to physical education and mental deficiency were studied. In the inaugural speech, Martínez Vargas explained the problem of infant mortality. In Spain at that time, for every 100 deaths, 45.53% were children from nought to ten years old. Motivated by this situation he wrote: *"The preferential attention dedicated to children, the desire that exists everywhere to protect their lives, to make them healthy, strong and happy, to help them avoid cruel punishments, and to lighten the effort needed for their instruction, is a modern and surprising initiative: How have so many centuries been allowed to pass without caring for children and how have we had the indifference to see them die in numbers? In view of today's pressures, one might say that society, remorseful of the neglect of children until the end of the last century, is now hastening to make up for lost time, to recapture the abandoned beneficent trenches"*. But Martínez Vargas was also worried about the serious problem at that time due to the reduction in the birthrate. As a result, decades before other authors, he presented a series of measures that had to be implemented for improved parenting and better education. Firstly he discussed preconception childcare and said that *"one of the measures would be the medical marriage license, or in other words, eugenic marriage"*. Here we see a glimpse of genetic counselling, even at the beginning of the twentieth century.

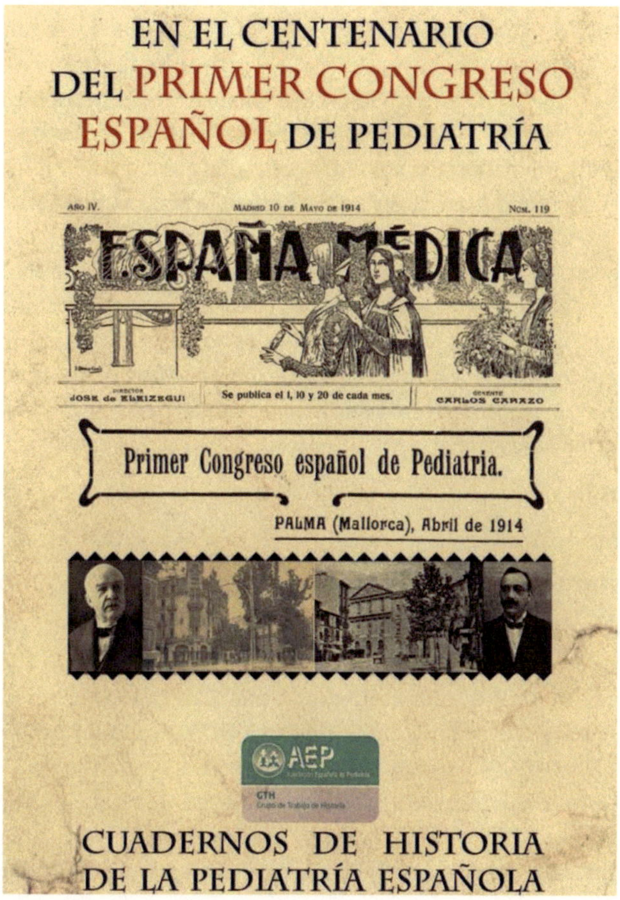

Figure 15. Cuadernos de historia de la pediatría española. Given permission from AEP

He later advocated embryonic and foetal childcare, which saw the start of Prenatal Medicine, arguing for all kinds of care that the mother should receive from the moment of conception, insisting on the need for joint medical care for the pregnant woman and the unborn child. His interest in the care of pregnant women is shown when he writes: *"The working woman, who has to split the hours in the day between the factory and the home, has two great enemies to the strength and vitality of her child, namely excessive work and intoxications…, all those women who work tirelessly and are not adequately nourished give birth to children who weigh 300 grams less than others who enjoy rest and relaxation"*. He was also worried about single mothers: *"The helplessness of these mothers is a frequent cause of infanticide. It would be better, instead of wasting time in boards or meetings, to organise an asylum or shelter suitable for this pressing social need, where the mother could care for her child and later it could go to a nursery or preschool and the mother could return to the heart of society without boasting and without intimidation".* He insisted on the need for the government to oblige employers to install rooms in their factories where women could attend to and look after breastfeeding children, giving them the rest time needed. He anticipated current social advances by decades. He argued that before giving bottles of formula milk to children, the mother should be examined and provided with enough food to be able to breastfeed. He refused to accept that formula milk could replace a mother's milk. He rejected the idea that there were illnesses caused by children's drool, or that teething provoked fever, diarrhoea or bronchitis. The minutes and papers from the congress are a monument to the paediatrics of the day. Martínez Vargas collaborated decisively in writing the conclusions, among which the highlights include those regarding childcare and child protection by the State. He argued that this must distribute the mother's code so that its advice could be followed, prohibit contraception propaganda, promulgate the law on rest for pregnant women, giving them two months' rest, stimulate the spreading of child protection policies, encourage breastfeeding, control the industry "originated around wet nurses" and that of the manufacture of bottles, reward families with more than three living children, impose a tax on celibacy, in the Teaching Schools child care should be explained, minors should be protected through the appropriate laws…" *Protect children for being the joy of every home, the comfort of old age…the vitality of the nation…Without them nations would disappear"*

20. The encounter with doctor Fidel Pagés Miravé, discoverer of the epidural anaesthetic

There is a chapter of the life of our protagonist that demonstrates his future vision. After reading the article "*Anestesia Metamérica*" (Metameric Anaesthesia) by the military surgeon Fidel Pagés Miravé (1886-1923), born in Huesca, he invited him to the University of Barcelona to discuss his discovery. The aforementioned Doctor Alfredo Cebrián wrote a footnote in pencil on the Treatise by Comby: "*Yesterday, 4 March 1922, I attended, with students, physicians and surgeons, an interesting talk given by Doctor Fidel Pagés about a new form of anaesthesia. It was held in a paediatrics classroom and we attendees were very impressed, applauding enthusiastically after the speech was over. Andrés closed the brilliant event*".

Doctor Pagés described his technique in these words: " …*On performing a spinal anaesthesia, I had the idea of stopping the cannula right in the spinal canal, before going through the dura mater, and I proposed blocking the roots outside the meningeal space, before going through the intervertebral foramina, given that the tip of the needle had gone through the corresponding ligamentum flavum. I abandoned the anaesthetic that I had prepared, and in a boiled capsule I made the dissolution of three tablets of series A suprarenine novocaine (375 milligrams of novocaine) in 25 cubic centimetres of saline solution, immediately injecting it through the cannula, which was embedded between the second and third lumbar vertebrae. Exploring sensitivity, we could convince ourselves that after five minutes a hypoesthesia began in the infra-umbilical portion of the abdomen, which extended to the anterolateral*

http://dx.doi.org/10.5772/58889

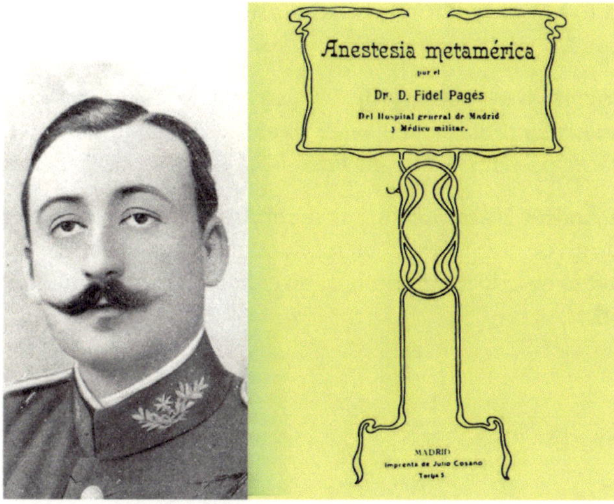

Figure 16. Dr. Fidel Pagés Miravé and the cover of his epidural anaesthesia article. Found out in Julio Comby paediatric treatise

side of the lower limbs leaving the perineum, scrotum, back side of the lower limbs and the soles of the foot on both sides untouched; the hyperaesthesia gained strength gradually, and twenty minutes after the injection had been give we judged it appropriate to start operating, performing a miracle cure of the right inguinal hernia without any discomfort to the patient. The result of this attempt encouraged us to continue studying this method, which in the clinic we call metameric anaesthesia, since it gives us the possibility of removing feeling from a segment of the body…" He then explained that his experience in this type of anaesthesia exceeded two hundred patients. His article was published in the *Revista Española de Cirugía* (Spanish Journal of Surgery) in 1921, which he had founded two years earlier. Despite his premature death, he operated on more than two thousand patients using this original anaesthetic technique.

Andrés Martínez Vargas suspected that this discovery would revolutionise the world of anaesthesiology. He also agreed with Fidel Pagés that it could be applied to women during childbirth. Today it is known as Epidural Anaesthesia. Fidel Pagés Miravé is not sufficiently recognised, either in Spain or internationally, despite his brilliance [24]. The history of his discovery, of the alleged claim by another foreign physician to have invented this technique, his short life which ended in a fatal car accident, and his scant subsequent recognition, require a specific article. Officially he is considered the discoverer of the epidural anaesthesia.

21. Conclusions

This information about Martínez Vargas, despite being the result of reading and analysing most of his work, is not exhaustive and may be supplemented.

The impression one gets when looking at the work of Martínez Vargas is of his interest and curiosity about medicine, art, humanism, sociology, his love for children, his desire to serve

Spain, and his wish to not only improve health care levels but also help society as a whole advance.

At his death the following was written [10]: *"He was extolled and widely acclaimed… He also knew what humility, intrigue, ingratitude and slander meant… A magnificent professor, an exceptional physician and a terrific man… He lived for his three great ideals, science, his homeland and children"*

I firmly believe that Andrés Martínez Vargas deserves the recognition of his countrymen and the scientific world, given the interest of his works and the wonderful complexity of his character. There is yet to be a doctoral thesis or an exhaustive study made about his passionate life and his vast works.

Acknowledgements

Professor Serafín Málaga Guerrero, President of the Spanish Paediatric Association, for his tireless work representing Spanish paediatricians; to Professor Eduardo G. Pérez-Yarza, for his friendship and work in favour of the speciality; to Professor Empar Lurbe i Ferrer, Chief Editor of "Anales de Pediatría"; to to Professor Manuel Bueno Sánchez, President of Royal Academy of Medicine and Surgery of Zaragoza; to Professor Juan Rodríguez Soriano (1933-2010), eminent paediatric nephrologist, discoverer of Renal tubular acidosis, magister of several paediatricians and nephrologists; Doctor Nuria García Sánchez, president of the Aragon, La Rioja and Soria Paediatric Association, for the same reason; to Dr. Víctor García Nieto, a great paediatric nephrologist, history expert and friend; to Doctor Juan Elías, President of paediatric surgeons of Spain; to Alejandro Labay Guerrero, my little son, for his help with ofimatics.

Author details

Miguel Labay Matías*

Address all correspondence to: mlabaymatias@hotmail.com, mlabay@salud.aragon.es

University of Zaragoza, Health Sciences, University School of Nursing in Teruel, Government of Aragon, HEALTH, Spain

References

[1] Labay Matías M. Andrés Martínez Vargas: un médico distinto nacido en Barbastro. Apuntes humanos de su vida. En: El Cruzado Aragonés. Barbastro (ed.); Agosto, 2012. p7-15.

[2] Labay Matías M. Jerónimo Soriano y Andrés Martínez Vargas: dos pilares aragoneses de la pediatría española. En: Turia. Revista cultural. Instituto estudios turolenses, Diputación Provincial Teruel 104(ed.) Teruel; 2012. p353-362.

[3] Labay Matías M. Pediatría, ciudadanos y políticos. An Pediatr (Barc). 2010; 73 (2) 67-69.

[4] Gómez Pano, JR, Espina Capo A, Martínez Vargas A. La oficina de farmacia española. Suplementos séptimo-duodécimo. Madrid: Baylly-Baylliere, (ed.); 1887-1895.

[5] Martínez Vargas A. Prólogo. En: Amargós Bertrán L. Estados Unidos. Viaje de un turista curioso. Madrid: Hesperia (ed.); 1947.

[6] Labay Matías M. Paediatrics, the people and politicians in Spain-History, development, reality and future. In: Contemporary Pediatrics, Dr. Öner Özdemir. Rijeka: In Tech. 2012. p1-24.http://www.intechopen.com/articles/show/title/pediatrics-the-people-and-politicians-in-spain-history-development-reality-and-future (accessed 7 July 2014).

[7] Fleta Zaragozano J., editor. Los pediatras y la pediatría aragonesa a finales del siglo XIX y principios del XX. Su relación con el entorno social de la época. Sesión de clausura del curso1987-88 de la Sociedad de Pediatría de Aragón, La Rioja y Soria. Zaragoza: Artes Gráficas Impr.; 1988.

[8] Martínez Vargas A., editor. Tratado de Pediatría. Barcelona: J. Vives, Tip. Lit. (ed.); 1915.

[9] Martínez Vargas A. El Ministerio de Sanidad en España. Real Academia de Medicina y Cirugía. Acta sesión conmemorativa del tercer cincuentenario, celebrada el 29 de diciembre de 1920. Barcelona Joaquín Horta, Impr. (ed.); 1921.

[10] Samper Villagrasa P. Andrés Martínez Vargas: semblanza de un pediatra ilustre. Available in: Dialnet.unirioja.es/servlet: (accessed 3 July 2014); 2004.

[11] Martínez Vargas A. Traducción y comentarios. En: Comby J. Enfermedades de la infancia. 3ª edición. Barcelona: Salvat é hijo (ed.); 1901.

[12] Labay Matías M, Valle Sánchez F, Reynés Muntaner J, Gómez Rivas B, Hervás Palazón J, Moros Peña M. Red de fibrina en líquido cefalorraquídeo de los niños con meningitis tuberculosa: un antiguo, olvidado y eficaz método para su diagnóstico precoz. An Esp Pediatr 2000; 53 (5) 502-503.

[13] Unger L editor. Tratado de las Enfermedades de los niños. Tercera y Cuarta Edición. Barcelona: José Espasa (ed.); 1899.

[14] Martínez Vargas, A. Botiquín escolar. Publicaciones de la escuela moderna. Segunda edición. Barcelona: Elveriziana, Borrás y Mestre, Impr (ed.); 1908.

[15] Martínez Vargas A. Tratamiento de la Fiebre tifoidea con el Suero. Publicaciones de la Medicina de los niños. Barcelona: Jaime Vives, Establ. Tip. (ed.); 1910.

[16] Martínez Vargas A. En defensa de la raza. Discurso. Apertura curso académico de 1918 a 1919. Universidad de Barcelona. Barcelona: La Académica de Serra y Rusell, Tip. (ed.); 1918.

[17] García Nieto V., y Grupo de historia y documentación pediátricas de la Asociación Española de Pediatría. Historia de la Pediatría española de Martínez Vargas A. Reedición. En Crónicas de la pediatría española. Tenerife: Asociación Española de Pediatría; 2011.

[18] Martínez Vargas A. Mi visita al frente Francés. Barcelona: J. Vives Tip. (ed.); 1919.

[19] Soriano J. Methodo, y orden de curar las enfermedades de los niños. Prólogos de Arana Amurrio JI, Sarabia Pardo J. Facsímil. Granada: Alhulia (ed.); 2000.

[20] Martínez Vargas A. La salud del niño. Consejos a las madres para la mejor crianza de sus hijos. Sociedad Lechera Montañesa. Barcelona: Nagsa (ed.); 1947.

[21] O'Neill E. Prólogo de Martínez Vargas A. La voz humana. Barcelona: Maucci (ed.); 1921.

[22] Labay Matías M. Pueribus. Finalista I Certamen nacional relatos breves. Real Academia de Medicina y Cirugía. Murcia: Org Art Gráf. Churra (ed.); 2011.

[23] Libro-Actas I Congreso Nacional Pediatría. Palma de Mallorca: Escuela Tipográfica Provincial (ed.): 1915.

[24] Labay Matías M. Andrés Martínez Vargas. En: Asociación Española de Pediatría (ed.) En el Centenario del Primer Congreso Español de Pediatría. Cuadernos de Historia de la Pediatría Española, número 7. Tenerife: Asociación Española de Pediatría;2014. p20-30.

[25] Ponte F, Zafra M, Fernández JM, Gorrotxategui P, Bassat Q, Fernández JJ, Arana JI, García Nieto V. Tal como éramos. En el centenario del Primer Congreso Español de Pediatría de Palma de Mallorca (1914-2014). An Pediatr (Barc). 2014;80(6): 404.e1-408.e8.http://dx.doi.org/10.1016/j.anapedi.2014.03.010 (accessed 7 July 2014).

[26] Velázquez Rivera I. Aproximación a la obra científica del Comandante médico Fidel Pagés Miravé. Sanid. Mil. 2011; 67 (1): 193-238.jhttp://scielo.isciii.es/scielo.php?script=sci_arttext&pid=S1887-85712011000300003&lng=es. http://dx.doi.org/10.4321/S1887-85712011000300003 (accessed 6 July 2014)

Section 2

Nursing Issues

Chapter 2

A Nursing Approach to Food Allergies

Şenay Çetinkaya

Additional information is available at the end of the chapter

http://dx.doi.org/10.5772/59320

1. Introduction

It is known for more than 2000 years that foods give rise to negative reactions in the body. The first unexpected reaction of the body due to foods is the reaction to the cow's milk, as defined by Hippocrates [1,2]. In 1921, Prausnitz and Kustner defined the allergic reaction, for the first time, with their fish allergy model [2]. They injected the serum of the individual with fish allergy into the insensitized individual, after which they formed an edema plaque by applying the serum intradermally [1].

Single-blind placebo-controlled food challenge (SBPCFC) studies were released for the first time in 1950, while double-blind placebo-controlled food challenge (DBPCFC) studies were released in 1976 [1].

The incidence of allergies has become a matter of concern for the last 50 years throughout the world. Although the reason for this is the research subject of separate scientific fields, it has been quite important to define this ailment and to inform people about such a condition that has become sort of an epidemic today [3].

Even in England, where the social welfare level and the average level of consciousness / awareness are higher than the values in our country, the public awareness for the matter involved had not developed before the beginning of 1990s. In those years, the several ensuing deaths, the cause of which was based on food allergy, had drawn much of the media's attention. In the wake of those tragic deaths, the public opinion urged the government to take action on the matter, and within a short time, an alarming situation showed up in the food industry. On the same dates, about a thousand people came together under the roof of the institution called *Anaphylaxis Campaign* to share their experiences and to find out solutions to this situation. According to the records of that time, the majority of the patients consisted of children aged 15 at most (80%), whereas the nutrient that was complained most about was the peanut (85%). In the face of these figures, the English officials prompted the involved ministries and the government agencies to take action for the purpose of carrying out researches and launching preventive programs. The records kept by the non-governmental organizations (NGO) during that time and the surveys performed so far give us information as to the course of these ailments [3].

Food allergy is defined as the reactions of the human body against food proteins, which occur through immunological mechanisms [4,5].

The prevalence of food allergy is associated with age and diet [2,5]. The incidence of food allergies has increased incrementally in recent years [4]. It is seen more frequently in the early years of a lifetime [2]. The burden of food allergy in the pediatric clinics is on the increase [6]. This ailment is seen in 6% of children and in 3-4% of adults [4]. Its prevalence in childhood occurs with the highest incidence in the early years of life [6]. On the other hand, the prevalence of food allergy among the those with atopic eczema (atopic dermatitis) is around 35% [1], while the food additive sensitivity in children is reported to be 0.5-1% [1].

The Center for Disease Control and Prevention (CDC) reported that the food allergy in children increased at a rate of 18% between 1997-2007 and that 3.9% of the children were affected by this ailment [2].

A systematic review by RAND Corp was performed by using pre specified criteria directed toward obtaining articles on epidemiological aspects of food allergy and resulted in the conclusion that food allergy affected from 1% to 2% up to 10% of the population [5]. Branum and Lukacs reported that in 2007, on the basis of the National Health Interview Survey response to the query, "During the past 12 months has [child] had any kind of food or digestive allergy?"3.9% of US children were affected [5,7].

In the study where the children with food allergy who applied to HUMF (Hacettepe University, Medical Faculty), Children's Allergy&Asthma Unit between 2002-2007 were incorporated in the study with respect to the prevalence of food allergy, it was determined that the kids under the age of 1 were mostly allergic to cow's milk and eggs, whereas those aged 1 and above were allergic to hazelnut-peanut-walnut, meat, legumes (chickpea, lentil, peas) and fish [4]. In Adana, the incidence of cow's milk allergy until the age of 1 was found to be 1.5% [1]. While the great majority of early childhood food allergies, such as cow's milk, eggs, wheat and soy, clear up until the school age, 80% of peanut, fish and shellfish allergies continue throughout lifetime [4,8]. Besides the fact that the type of the nutrient is important in developing tolerance to nutrients, the genetic risk factors, such as an atopic disease within the family, and the factors like environmental and cultural dietary habits play a clinical role in the occurrence of food allergies [4,5,7-10].

The prevalence of food allergies has been on a continual increase in recent years [4,7]. A study conducted in the USA has suggested that the peanut allergy in children has doubled within five years. According to the routine patient records in England, the incidence of anaphylaxis has increased 7 times more, while the food allergy increased 5 times more during the past 10 years. It was shown that 56% of those with anaphylaxis treated in the emergency departments in Australia were due to food allergy [4]. These conclusions clearly show that food allergy is a significant public health concern [6]. Today food allergies in the western countries are regarded as a public health issue [4].

Foods may cause many various undesirable reactions and diseases, which may sometimes be fatal [4,7]. Almost 20% of the society change their diets due to an undesirable reaction developing against foods. These undesirable reactions occur due to an immunological response to a food protein (e.g. food allergy), a metabolic disease (e.g. lactose intolerance, galactosemia), pharmacological response (e.g. nervousness due to caffeine, headache due to thyramine within cheese) or toxic reactions (e.g. bacterial food poisoning) [4].

In 2001, The European Academy of Allergy and Clinical Immunology (EAACI) reclassified the hypersensitivity reactions due to foods according to their pathogeneses. All the non-toxic harmful food reactions observed after the intake of foods/nutrients were referred to as **food hypersensitivity**. If the reaction occurred through an immunological mechanism, then the term, '**food allergy**' was used, and if the presence of IgE was shown, then the term, "**IgE-mediated food allergy**" was used. The reactions also defined previously as the food intolerance were named as the **non-allergic food hypersensitivity** [4]. Although each nutrient may cause a reaction, a few nutrients are partially responsible for most of the important allergic food reactions, which can be sorted as milk, eggs, types of nuts, peanut, fish and shellfish [4]. The most allergic foods in children are the cow's milk, eggs, nut, peanut, fish and tomatoes [1].

Food Allergens: The factors giving rise to food allergens despite the consumption of many varieties of foods are generally limited in number. Food allergens are grouped in 2 classes [4].

First Class Allergens: These are the main sensitizing allergens, and the most important food allergens fall within this group [4]. Resistant to heat, acid and protease, food allergens are the water-soluble substances with a glycoprotein structure, the molecule weight of which is 10-60 kD [1,4].

The allergic reaction to these foods/nutrients develops after the oral food intake. The cow's milk, eggs, peanut, soy, shrimps and lipid transfer proteins (apple, apricot, peach, plum, corn) fall within this group [4].

The Second Group of Allergens, on the other hand, are mostly vegetative proteins (profilins). Since their temperature-sensitive structures can be easily spoiled, it is difficult to isolate and keep them for a long time. Most of the vegetative allergens within this group show a structural similarity to the proteins associated with the pathogens in most pollens, profilins, peroxidases and peroxidase inhibitors [4].

Any nutrient can be an allergen. The cow's milk is a significant allergen during childhood which provides the earliest finding in this matter. There are at least 20 proteins in a cow's milk, the most important allergenic protein of which is the Beta lactoglobulin (β-Lactoglobulin). It is of a more allergenic character when compared with the egg white (albumen) or egg yolk (duetoplasm). The ovomucoid in the egg white (Gal d 1) is the most important allergen of all. The other egg allergens are ovalbumin (Gal d 2), ovotransferrin (Gal d 3) and lysozyme (Gal d 4) [1].

Severe or fatal food anaphylaxis can be seen at any age, even in the first confrontation with the nutrient. However, the adolescents with asthma or young adults who allergic to peanuts, hazelnuts and sea products are at greatest risk in terms of fatal food anaphylaxis. The incidence of food allergies is associated with age. In the USA, food allergy was determined in 8% of the kids under the age of three, 6% of those in their school age and in 3.7% of the adults. The types of food that cause allergies most frequently are also associated with age. In the USA, the most common allergies determined in little kids were those related with the cow's milk (2.5%), eggs (1.3%), peanut (0.8%), wheat (0.4%), soy (0.4%), tree nuts (0.2%) and fish (0.1%). The allergies related with shellfish (2%), peanut (0.6%) and fish (0.1%) are seen in adults more often. The reactions to fruit and vegetables are also common with approximately 0.5%; yet, these reactions are usually not serious. Seed allergies, such as sesame, are reported to be seen more and more frequently [4]. It seems that the sesame seed will be recognized more and more in terms of allergies [11].

The allergic diseases triggered by foods/nutrients occur through the pathway of cell-mediated reactions that cause an acute or subacute inflammation through medium of the pathway of food-specific IgE antibodies and the activation of the effector cells, or through the simultaneous activation of the effector cells by both of the pathways [4].

1.1. The conditions in which cross-reactivity is observed among food allergies in clinics and the cross-reactivity risks

1. **Among the Botanical Families:**

    - Legumes: Reaction Risk for another legume is 5%.
    - Cereals: Tahıllar: Reaction Risk for another cereal is 20%.
    - Tree Nuts: Reaction Risk for another type of nut is 37%.
    - The Risk of Cross-Reaction among Rosaceae Fruits is 55%.

2. **Among the Types of Food:**

    - Fish: Reaction Risk for another type of fish is 50%.
    - The Reaction Risk among Shellfish is 75%.
    - Cow's Milk: Reaction Risk for bovine meat is 10%, while it is 92% for goat's milk.

3. **Food/Nutrient-Pollen:** The Reaction Risk for any fruit/vegetable through pollen allergy is 55%.

    - Birch Tree: Apple, carrot, cellery, raw Potato, chestnut.
    - Grass: Tomato, potato, cherry, peach.
    - Ragweed: Melon, Banana.
    - Artemisia: Cellery, apple, peanut, kiwi.

4. **Food/Nutrient-Non-Pollen:**

    - Latex allergy: Reaction Risk for Fruits (banana, chestnut, avocado, kiwi) is 35%.

http://dx.doi.org/10.5772/59320

- Fruit allergy: Reaction Risk for Latex is 11% [4].

Foods/Nutrients produce various symptoms in the cutaneous, gastrointestinal and respiratory systems through IgE-mediated and Non-IgE (cellular) mechanisms [4,12]. There are still several studies conducted in order to figure out how the normal oral tolerance disfunctions and the food allergy occurs [4].

The mucosal barrier in the gastrointestinal system, enzymes, peyer's plaques in the intestinal wall, cells providing antigens and T and B cells have a significant role in the development of food allergies. On the other hand, there is the intestinal/bowel barrier which hinders the development of food allergies, and there are mechanisms referred to as oral tolerance, which prevent the development of immune response to food antigens in the bowel [4].

The intestinal flora is formed within the first 24 hours of life and remains stable throughout lifetime; the maternal flora is dependent on genetic and local environment [4].

Food allergies occur in the genetically susceptible individuals as the result of the failure of the oral tolerance to develop normally or the disfunctioning of the oral tolerance [4]. Food allergy reactions are described by Gell-Coombs Hypersensitivity Reaction; however, food hypersensitivity is a much more complicated reaction [1]. In food allergies, not only the humoral immune response but also the cellular mechanisms play a significant role [4,12]. Type I hypersensitivity reaction develops through **IgE**. As the result of the dysfunctioning of oral tolerance or its failure to develop, **specific IgE antibodies are performed within the nutrient**, and they join the high-affinity receptor, FceR1 in **the mast cell** and **basophils**, or the low-affinity receptors on the **monocyte**, **macrophage**, **lymphocyte** and **eosinophil**. Food allergens reach the antibody that passes through the mucosal barrier and joins the fab section. In consequence of this connection, the mast cell is activated; histamine, prostaglandin and leukotrienes are released, and these released/oscillated mediators lead to vasodilatation, smooth muscle contraction and mucus secretion in various tissues and organs. This is the early hypersensitivity reaction, which takes place within minutes. From this activated mast cell, various cytokines, such as **IL-4, IL-5, IL-6, IL-13 and PAF** are released/oscillated, which produce a **late allergic reaction of IgE origin**. **Neutrophiles and eosonophiles reach the scene in 4-8 hours**. The mediators, including PAF, bring about the release/oscillation of peroxidase, ECP and EBP. **Lymphocytes and monocytes are responsible for the chronic inflammation that occurs within 24-48 hours.** Some part of the nutrient-based reactions is the food hypersensitivity of non-IgE origin [1].

Th2 phenotype is found in atopic patients and the IL-4, IL-5, IL-13 and IgE antibody formations against unknown proteins increase [2].

1.2. The classification of food allergies

Food allergies are classified according to the immunological mechanisms and the involvement of the organ systems playing a role in the process [4,10].

IgE-mediated food allergies with acute onset:		
	Skin: Rash (Urticaria), angioedema, morbilliform skin eruption/rash and flush in the face.	
	Gastrointestinal: Oral allergy syndrome, gastrointestinal anaphylaxis.	
	Respiration: Acute rhinoconjunctivitis, bronchospasm (wheezing)	
	Generalized: Anaphylactic shock.	
IgE associated/cell-mediated, late-onset/chronic food allergies:		
	Skin: Atopic dermatitis	
	Gastrointestinal: Allergic eosinophilic esophagitis/gastritis/gastroenteritis	
	Respiration: Asthma	
Cellular-mediated, late-onset/ chronic food allergies:		
	Skin: Contact Dermatitis, dermatitis herpetiformis	
	Gastrointestinal: Food Protein Enterocolitis	
		Food protein proctocolitis
		Food protein-induced enteropathy syndromes
		Celiac Disease
	Respiration: Pulmonary hemosiderosis (Heiner's syndrome)[4].	

Today a number of allergens contained within the nutriens/foods have been defined on a molecular level and synthesized. The immunopathogenesis of food allergies have been understood better, as the result of which new approaches of diagnosis and treatment can be put forward soon [4,13].

2. Food allergy clinic

An allergic reaction occurs in various organs through the foods/nutrients taken in, the most severe form of which is anaphylaxis. There may be atopic dermatitis, rash, angioedema, flushing and itching on the skin; while in the gastrointestinal system, swelling in the lips, tongue and palate, flushness, oropharyngeal edema, laryngeal edema, vomiting, diarrhea, upper and lower respiratory tract problems, wheezing, coughing and nasal congestion can be seen [1].

As the result of the food allergy, the following clinical symptoms can occur, apart from the condition of anaphylaxis [14] :

Digestive system:

- In-mouth sores
- Itching on the lips, tongue, palate and throat, sense of tickling, metallic taste
- Swelling in the lips and tongue

http://dx.doi.org/10.5772/59320

- Hoarseness
- Sense of jamming/congestion in the throat
- Nausea, vomiting
- Cramps
- Abdominal Distension
- Diarrhea, greasy-mucus (slimy) excrement/stool
- Bloody Excrement/Stool
- Constipation
- Gastro-oesophageal reflux

Skin:

- Itching
- Rush, hot flush
- Itchy/Scratchy water-logged rashes
- Swelling in the eyes, hands and feet
- Rash (Urticaria)
- Allergic Eczema

Respiratory system:

- Nasal Congestion, itching, sneezing, nasal flow
- Warbling in the throat (Stridor)
- Coughing
- Wheezing in the chest
- Sense of chest tightness, shortness of breath (dyspnea)
- Asthma

Eyes:

- Itching and watering of the eyes.

Systemic:

- Anaemia
- Loss of appetite (anorexia)
- Retardation in growth and development, loss of weight
- Decrease in Blood Pressure

- Black-out / Loss of consciousness, fainting.

There may be clues as to whether the food is taken in outside home or when it is taken in. For instance, egg rings in an Asian restaurant may contain eggs, peanuts and/or shrimps. The cross-contamination potential of the foods consumed in snack bars, ice cream shops and bakery/ patisseries is quite high [11].

The Second Disease Along with the Major One: The risk of developing food allergy in young children with atopic dermatitis is higher, particularly more serious and resistant to treatment, than that in the babies and those with intracutaneous reactivity in the toddler period. In general, the factors that may cause food allergy in younger patients and in those with more severe atopic dermatitis are more likely to be seen [11].

In particular, the food diaries in chronic patients would be of help in terms of their medical history [4]. Therefore, the patients should be allowed to keep diet diaries [1], in which the patient should note whatever s/he eats and drinks, along with the time of intake. In addition, they should also point out the type of the symptoms, and when and how often they occur in those diaries. If several distinct problems pop out, they should pick out two or three of the symptoms perceived as the worst ones. This may generally require a few weeks to perform [14].

The clinical history is of great value in acute food reactions (anaphylaxia, urticaria, etc.). On the other hand, this value in the chronic cases, such as atopic dermatitis, asthma and eosinophilic gastroenteritis, is rather low [1].

In the physical examination, the focus should be directed to the cutaneous, gastro-intestinal and respiratory systems, and atopic findings should also be sought [1].

After having acquired the medical record carefully to establish a diagnosis, the diagnosis is finalized through the laboratory studies, elimination diets and food provocation tests later on [4].

In fact, when double-blind placebo-controlled food challenge (DBPCFCs) is used in the diagnosis of IgE-mediated food allergy, the diagnoses of almost 40% of the nutrient-based reactions which were likely to be in various forms in the past could be verified [11].

While the possibility of the positive skin test to indicate food allergy in a patient is less than 50%, the possibility of the negative nutrient/food allergy test to indicate no food allergy in a patient is 95% [1].

Other similar in vitro studies, including RAST and ELISA, are significant scanning methods to determine the reactions of IgE origin in the serum, specific to the allergens but less sensitive than the skin test. RAST test should be preferred to the skin test in those with positive dermographism, in the patients regularly taking antihistaminics and in those with severe skin disease [1].

The elimination diet is used for the purpose of diagnosis and treatment. When an acute reaction (such as rash and anaphylaxis) caused by nutrients occurs, the nutrient in question has to be immediately eliminated from the diet. The remission of the reaction and the positive outcome of the skin test through that nutrient indicate that the nutrient in question plays a role in this reaction. In elimination, the growth of the baby should be followed-up with great care. When,

http://dx.doi.org/10.5772/59320

in milk elimination, there is recovery through diet, then the lactose intolerance should also be taken into consideration. The oral food challenge test is a major method of diagnosis in the identification and diagnosis of food allergy, which is performed in 3 ways:

1. Open; the doctor and the patient have the knowledge of the loaded food content.
2. Single-blind placebo-controlled; the patient is not informed about the loaded food content, except for the doctor him/herself.
3. Double-blind placebo-controlled; neither the doctor nor the patient knows anything about the content of the loaded substance [1].

3. Prognosis

The clinical tolerance in some foods (milk, eggs, soy, wheat) may develop more frequently than that in the others (peanut, tree fruits, sea products). In the former studies, the tolerance rate for milk and eggs between the ages 3 and 5 was reported to be 80%. More recent retrospective studies put forward in the study from John Hopkins Pediatric Allergy Clinic the resolution rate of those aged 16 with cow's milk allergy as 79% and the resolution rate of those aged 16 with egg allergy as 68%. This generalization may not be reflective on the society since there are also academic centers full of patients with more severe conditions, who are more resistant to the disease. On the other hand, almost 20% of little kids develop tolerance against the peanut, and less than 10% of them recover from the tree nut allergy [11].

4. The treatment

The most important method in food allergy is the elimination. The elimination diets may lead to malnutrition, and nutrition and eating disorders, thus, great care must be taken in this matter and a proper nutrient must be replaced with the one in question. Yet, some problems are confronted when more than one food allergy occur. The medications used in the treatment are antihistaminics (H1, H2), ketotifen, cromolyn sodium, corticosteroids, and prostaglandin synthetase inhibitors. Adrenaline becomes a life-saving factor when needed. It is used in the oral corticosteroid chronic reaction of IgE origin (atopic dermatitis, asthma) and in gastroenteritis of non-IgE origin (allergic eosinophilic esophagitis, gastroenteritis, the enteropathies occurring through diet). The oral chromolyn is used in the IgE-origin food allergy and allergic eosinophilic gastroenteritis, however, its efficiency has not been fully put forth [1].

The ability to identify the common allergens in the commercially prepared USA foods has become easy thanks to the laws in effect. *Food Allergen Labeling and Consumer Protection Act* (*FALCPA*) (by January 2006) (milk, eggs, soy, wheat, peanut, tree nuts, fish and shellfish) makes it obligatory for the substances derived from the common allergic sources to be labelled in English [11].

5. The self-injectable epinephrine (Adrenaline) indications

Children diagnosed with food allergy carry the risk of an immediate reaction once they are exposed to an allergic nutrient [8]. Since anaphylaxis may develop in the wake of the allergen exposure, it is advised that the patients be prescribed an epinephrine auto-injector in order to be able to do it by themselves, because the antihistaminics do not prevent the systemic reaction. In particular, it should be administered to those with the risk of developing fatal food anaphylaxis and to those with asthma and/or those suffering from tree nuts, such as peanut or hazelnut [10,15].

Epinephrine is a method of treatment clearly preferred for anaphylaxis. It was introduced and recognized in 2006 and was then put on the market. If there is any doubt of exposure to an allergen, then epinephrine should be applied in the event that an allergic reaction occurs right after two or more exposures (within a few minutes or a few hours) stated below :

- Skin or Mucosal Involvement (e.g. Common rash (urticaria) or the swelling or blistering of the oral mucosa.)
- The risk of Inadequate Respiration (e.g. Dyspnea, wheezing, stridor).
- Permanent gastro-intestinal symptoms (e.g. Vomiting).
- Hypotension (e.g. Hypotony, syncope). [10].

Undoubtedly, an epinephrine application and administration is an indication in a kid known with his/her hypotension symptoms (and even without accompanying symptoms) and food allergy in particular. When indicated, epinephrine is injected intramuscularly, preferably on the lateral of the femur. The plasma concentration of the high peak value of epinephrine/ adrenaline was demonstrated by the injection into vastus lateralis when compared to the deltoid. Moreover, the adrenaline plasma peak time concentration is 8±2 minutes after injection, however, it takes much longer (34±14 minutes) after the subcutaneous injection. The rapid administration of epinephrine is fundamental, since the respiratory or cardiac arrest period in those with anaphylaxis triggered by a nutrient is 30 minutes [15].

EpiPen and Twinject can both be used in two doses. The dose recommended for pediatric use is 0.01 mg/kg body weight. 0.3 mg dose is suitable for the patients close to 30 kg and above. The dose for the kids around 15 kg is indicated to be 0.15 mg. On the other hand, the clinical decision of the physician must be taken for the little kids (<10kg) and for those weighing between 15-30 kg [15].

When epinephrine is prescribed, it may appear to be non-applicable. However, the demonstration/ instruction of its application or training on it is a significant factor in encouraging patients for the use of epinephrine auto-injectors. The doctors are advised to demonstrate how to use these auto-injectors (preferably, via a placebo device) as well as giving verbal information [10,15].

The usual epinephrine dose is 0.01 mg/kg, and 0.5 mg (if required) at most can be repeated 5-30 minutes later. The approximate dose when the weight is unknown is 50 mcg (0.05 mL); for babies younger than 6 months, it is 120 mcg (0.12 mL); for those between 6 months and the age of 6, it is 250 mcg (0.25 mL), whereas the appropriate dose is 500 mcg (0.5 mL) for those aged between 6-12 and above. The injection must be performed intramuscularly through the femur. Training the health personnel and instructors in this matter is also necessary to avoid inadequate/partial use [6].

It has been estimated that food allergy and anaphylaxis alliance in USA is responsible for 200 deaths and 2000 hospitalizations in a year including but not limited to deaths and hospitalizations; 30.000 case for a year in all. The risk of anaphylaxis in children and the possibility of its recurrence due to a nutrient occur every other year, during which the attacks course with 0.6%-5 % mortality. With the diagnosis of food allergy, the anaphylaxis developing in children can be prevented. The deaths due to food anaphylaxis occur mainly away from home, and more public awareness for the matter involved will reduce the problem in question [6].

The pediatrician should perform 4 actions when the diagnosis of a possible fatal anaphylaxis is established:

- S/he should prescribe an epinephrine injector and describe how to and under what circumstances to use it.
- S/he should provide a plan of action in case of an emergency for the patient and the caregivers in the school, sports and other social activities.
- S/he should provide information as to the possibility of reaction occurrences and proper preventive and recovery measures.
- S/he should be advised to put an identification label on for a medical warning [6].

Antihistaminics, beta-agonists and systemic corticosteroids can be used as an adjuvant treatment for anaphylaxis. However, they should not be applied instead of epinephrine, since it has not yet been proved whether it reverses the respiratory or cardiovascular symptoms. Antihistaminics can be tried at the onset, and if the symptoms merely involve the skin (including the oral mucosa), the kid in question should be followed-up more closely in terms of the development of symptoms [15].

6. The prevention of atopy in brothers and sisters or children

Parents may often ask how they should prevent allergies in their children in the future. In 2008, the American Academy of Pediatrics (AAP) released a clinical report for the children with high-risk atopic development. The children with a high risk of allergy development were defined as: "There is a first-degree relative/relation (parents or brother/sister) with an allergic disease in the family circle of at least one of the children" [4]. The following suggestions are based on scientific facts and evidence in the prevention of food allergy and atopic dermatitis:

1. Breast-feeding for at least 4 months reduces the incidence of cow's milk allergy and atopic dermatitis in the first 2 years of life when compared with feeding on through the formula of cow's milk protein.
2. Atopic dermatitis can be held up or prevented with the common use of hydrolysis in early childhood or the partial use of hydrolized formulas when compared with the cow's milk formula within it. Common hydrolized formulas may partially be more effective than the partially hydrolized ones in terms of prevention, yet, the economic cost is significantly higher.
3. The soy-based formula has no role whatsoever in the prevention of allergy, and the amino acid formulas have not been studied in terms of preventing atopy.
4. Solid foods should not be taken in before 4-6 months. At this age, sufficient evidence lacks for dietary supplements at the time of intervention [15].

These suggestions are not valid for the patients whose atopic diseases like atopic dermatitis or food allergy have already developed [15].

There are a Few Problems in Diet Therapy:

- The child may be highly sensitive to the insignificant amount of food, and other modes of transmission must also be taken into account as some sort of substance used commonly in other foods may be the trigger for it.
- In addition to swallowing foods, skin contact and inhalation may lead to severe reactions; avoiding the external contacts and inhalation is generally essential.
- Cooking, especially at industrial nutrition, is a heat treatment process, raw food is able to been tolerated by sensitive person, so cooked (not raw) food avoidance may not be necessary in many cases.
- A simple elimination diet may be relative due to the fact that most of the allergic triggers and proteins of nutritional value can be found anywhere when the blameful food has been consumed [6].

Surprisingly, there are a few studies evaluating the effects of the elimination diet. The main concern of pediatricians may be the developmental delay in the children with allergies, particularly those with atopic dermatitis. According to a hypothesis, suppressing growth during infancy may indicate negative consequences in the years to come. Nevertheless, it is not yet clear whether the disease itself, the restricted diet, genetic factors or some combinations are the causes or not. Whatever the case may be, arranging the diet according to the babies and kids with food allergies require a more careful evaluation of the nutritional aspect on an individualistic basis. There is a consensus in the literature of food allergy, which is: " Extensive elimination diets need to be utilized only as a means for diagnosis for a short while.", and " It is quite important that a balanced diet containing proteins, calories, trace elements and vitamins be maintained.". This is particularly appropriate for the babies with cow's milk allergy. These babies should be provided with nutritional requirements, a balanced calorie-protein rate, aminoacid compound and adequate amount of calcium intake [6].

http://dx.doi.org/10.5772/59320

In most babies, the clinical reaction to foods ends once they reach their toddler period, thus, 90% of the babies with cow's milk allergy can tolerate milk towards the end of their 3rd years. However, half of their peers with egg allergy will not be able to get through to the same age. The peanut or codfish allergy in more than 80% of the patients still continue. The allergy or the food allergy perceived by parents may also be effective in the development of healthy nutritional habits. This transition period clinically requires the patients's review of avoidance strategy with his/her parents and periodic clinical revision of all the dietary interventions/attempts [6].

The American Academy of Allergy, Asthma & Immunology *(AAAAI),* Food Allergy Practice Parameters (2006) characterizes the immunotherapy for food allergy as "empirical" and states that it should be recognized as a clinical option. However, researches still continue, while the recombinant allergens or synthetic peptides appear to be more promising [6].

7. Labelling the processed foods

Labelling is a subject associated with food allergy, and it is the risk factor modified when the processed food, prior to packaging, is exposed to allergens by mistake. The laws in the European Union until recently did not give permission for the complicated contents listed on the labels on condition that they did not exceed 25% of all the products. Hence, the term "cremé" could be read on the label regardless of a clear indication of eggs as the combination of a sandwich/snack. Following the labelling guidelines in September 2001, this respect was extracted from the guideline in 2005. The law makes it a condition that the contents of 12 nutrients appear on the label: **eggs, peanut and tree nuts, soy, cow's milk (containing lactose), mustard, sesame seeds, cellery and the amount of sulfides more than 10 mg/kg**. Similar laws now effect the USA. In the beginning of 2006, Food Allergen Labeling and Consumer Protection Act makes it mandatory that the specifications for the ingredients be indicated on the labels of all food products. Once, the latent allergens were not labelled, since they were the additives free of the existing ingredients/specific labelling (e.g. Colour and aroma/flavor); however, if, from now on, they contain one of these 8 nutrients, they will need to be described then; therefore, most of the problems regarding the unlabelled/latent allergens in foods will be elimi*nated* [6].

8. Food allergy: Nutritional respects for the primary care providers

With the prominent increase in the prevalence of food allergy among children, the pediatricians must figure out how to follow-up the dietary status of these kids. Parents, particularly when the child requires a restricted diet, are typically dependent on the primary pediatrician in order to follow up their kid's growth and development. The role of an allergist is to provide the diagnosis and method for food allergy as well as the initial training and guidance. However, it may be beneficial to acquire further supportive and accurate information from the pediatrician who is often in contact with the family regarding inadequate nutrition and dietary management. A dietician experienced in food allergy and children can be an ideal person a family confers with; yet, this option may not be available in all the geographical regions [16].

9. The nutrition assessment in primary care

To date, the sole treatment for food allergy is to totally eliminate the food(s) that give rise to complaints. Potentially, due to the restrictive nature of avoiding any nutrient/food, the diagnosis method proven for the children with multi-food allergy in particular is quite important. If no reliable food allergy test has been performed or if it is restricted on the basis of the reports/information provided by parents or their own beliefs, the child may be at an unnecessary risk in terms of inadequate nutrition. Once a reliable test has been performed, the training on the foods to be avoided and foods in general should be provided, as the result of which the pediatrician can start the nutritional follow-up process [16].

10. Result

- Since the elimination of food products from the food may be both practically and nutritionally rather challenging, it is important that the diagnosis be established on an accurate basis.
- A distinction between the allergic reactions against food products and the hypersensitivity against nutritional compounds should be made.

Among the common food allergens are the peanut and tree nuts, egg white, sesame, cow's milk, legumes, soy, fish, shellfish and wheat. Although not directly, the consumption of other products in which these nutrients are added, or the products coming from the production line where those nutrients are processed cannot be considered clean in terms of allergy and unreliable/unhealthy for patients, towards which several countries are developing policies [3].

Food allergy has become a great social health issue throughout the world. With further awareness in the matter, the increase in the incidence is inevitable. Besides, the western pre-school nurseries, primary schools, secondary education institutions and public enterprises have constituted private programs and regulations to be able to cope with this issue [3,10].

The Responsibilities of Parents:

- To inform the school about the allergic condition of the student.
- To develop a plan to meet the requirements of the student within school, in the cafeteria, during the treatment in the wake of the disease, in school activities and in school service buses, etc. by working together with the school administration.
- To provide health documents, prescribed medications and the instructions for use as well as attaching the picture of the child to the involved folder.

- To supply accurately-labelled medications as well as renewing them after their usage and expiry date.
- To train the child in the subjects regarding food allergy as stated below:
- Safe and risky foods
- Preventive resorts/remedies for accessing risky foods.
- Symptoms of allergic reactions.
- The time and the way of informing the adults around about the developing allergic reaction.
- Reading the food labels.
- To review the current regulations or rules together with the school management, the physician responsible for the kid and the kid him/herself in the event that a reaction occurs.

To provide a contact info in case of an emergency [3,10].

The Responsibilities of A School:

- To have the knowledge of the involved regulations, and to have the capacity of perceiving and applying them correctly.
- To have already examined the health files from parents and physicians.
- To incorporate the students with food allergy in school activities.

To constitute a "preventive plan" by forming a skeleton crew consisting of a school nurse, a teacher, school manager, an administrator of food and nutritional services, and a school counselor and incorporating them in the food allergy management together with the student and his/her parents [3,10].

The Responsibilities of a Student:

- S/he shall not exchange foods with other students.
- S/he shall not consume foods with the content of allergens or foods with unknown content.
- S/he shall co-operate in the management of food allergy and in treatment processes.
- S/he shall immediately inform his/her family for the matter involved as soon as s/he realizes that s/he has consumed some food known to be allergic.
- Ultimately, the guidance provided by an allergist and a dietician, the association of allergic patients, and their feedback would increase the life quality of both the child and his/her parents.
- Further studies regarding the empowerment of children through training and the long-term impact of the elimination of a nutrient from the diet in terms of food allergy are required to be conducted.

The role of the pediatrician will have been fulfilled in this center with the suggestion made by a dietician [3,10].

11. Protection

Babies with the risk of atopy are those in whose family circle the mother, father or at least one of the brothers or sisters has a medical record of an atopic disease, such as asthma and allergic rhinitis [17].

As in all the health issues, protection is the leading approach in allergic diseases, as well. There are a number of studies researching into what could be done to prevent the disease in babies at risk, among which the protection from the allergens in the cow's milk has a significant place. The superiority of breast milk is indisputable in terms of both nutrition and protection. Thus, while the cow's milk or alternative diets are being discussed, they are always assessed according to breast milk. With quite an extensive cohort study about 70 years ago, Grulee and Sanford compared the babies fed on breast milk with those fed on mixed diet and suggested that the risk of eczema increased 9 times more with normal cow's milk [17].

Feeding a baby through breast milk prevents the development of an atopic disease. If an atopic heredity is involved, such a preventive feature becomes more prominent. If there is no breast milk or only an inadequate amount, a totally hydrolized baby food should be selected. Non-hydrolized or less hydrolized baby foods are risky in terms of atopy. It was seen that the risk of atopic dermatitis decreased at a rate of 50% in the first years of the lives of the babies at high risk who were fed on baby foods containing a totally hydrolized casein in the first 6 months [17].

Encouraging people in feeding babies who are at high risk and who have already food allergy through breast milk as well as other protective approaches and as early diagnosis and accurate treatment as possible are the steps to be taken for a healthy life-style [17,18].

12. Probiotics

Since human beings first existed on the Earth, they have been living with other creatures in an environment called the *nature*. The gastrointestinal system ensures the relationship of the human beings with the outer world. It is the inner side of us, but in fact, it is the outer side or the *universe* inside us. By taking the food and drink through our mouth, we send the bacteria that are the invisible creatures of the nature to our digestive system. Most of these bacteria are friendly bacteria. Those that survive the gastric acid, gall and pancreas enzymes continue their routes until the digestive system and connect or stick to the receptors there and start to live with us and become an integrated part of us [18].

These bacteria that ensure that we live healthily and protect ourselves from diseases and help us in treatments when they are taken in sufficient amounts are called PROBIOTIC BACTERIA. When the birth of a baby occurs via the vaginal method that is foreseen by the nature, the baby takes all the bacteria from the mother's colon and vagina flora through its mouth. These bacteria belong to the mother's flora and some of them (for example *Escherichia coli*) may be risky for the newborn. If the mother starts to breastfeed the child in the possible shortest time, the carbohydrates (prebiotics) in the form of galactose-oligo-saccharide that are existent in the mother's milk (i.e. prebiotics), are broken down by these bacteria. After this process, an energy coming from the short-chain fatty acids is obtained; and with this energy, the bacteria that are necessary for the child at that age-mainly the bifido-bacterium and lactobacillus group bacteria-start to grow in a fast pace (bifidogenic effect). At the end of the first week, the bifido-bacteria dominate in the 70-80% of the flora. The bacteria such as *E.coli* that may be risky for the child are suppressed and minimized in number [18].

Furthermore, essential fatty acids such as acetate, butyrate and propionate contribute to the development, in one sense, close the ranks of colonocites and enterocytes and prevent the migration of pathogen microorganisms and macromolecular foreign proteins from the lumen to the system. These essential fatty acids act as important energy sources for the functional development of the brain and liver [18].

Vaginal birth and the breast milk as soon as possible after the birth are the most important steps of the nature in the healthy life program of the human beings. Contrary to these steps, the babies who are born via caesarian method and/or the babies who cannot be fed with breast milk cannot start life in a heathy way, and these babies have relatively more allergic and inflammatory diseases [8,18,19].

13. The role of a nurse

In a nursing practice, the key role of a nurse is to provide consultancy, information and trust/security. A nurse provides information for the child, the youth and their families regarding other health issues, including the suspected type of allergy, its severity, the risk of an allergic reaction and the possible effects of a suspected allergy, on the basis of the allergy-oriented medical record of the child or the young patient [20].

A nurse, with a feasible plan, can also cover parents' lack of knowledge of the succeeding steps in achieving a final diagnosis that may involve the procedures of an elimination diet after performing skin tests and specific IgE antibody test. To provide adequate nutrition for babies and mothers, it is important that an awareness for requirement be maintained for alternative sources [20].

It cannot be expected of a nurse and/or a physician to become a specialist overnight on the diagnosis and management of allergy, considering the insufficient education and training provided for them in this matter. Nevertheless, it is crucial to become aware of the conditions to be suspected of food allergy and to take the necessary precautions in this respect [20].

Allergies are frequent, serious allergic reactions are less common, anaphylaxis is rare, so nurses should be aware of how to deal with anaphylaxis and management of these cases. More frequently, the primary care nurses will encounter children under such conditions as suspected allergy or the circumstances with an allergic component. The majority of those with an allergic disease can be cured in the first step/level, however, it is important that nurses and patients be in the know and aware of the local ways of referral in such applications [10,21].

14. Patient and/or parent training

Cow's milk allergy is the type of allergy which is most commonly seen in little children. What causes a reaction in the cow's milk allergy are the proteins within the milk. The treatment of milk allergy means the total removal of the milk. The milk obtained from goats, bisons and as such should also be avoided. Apart from what we refer to as the classic dairy products, the milk protein can be found in many food products, as well. Therefore, it is important to always read the product description very carefully in order to understand what products are safe to consume. It should also be kept in mind that the milk protein in the content list is defined sometimes as casein or curdled milk [22].

The substitutes for milk are the milk protein-based products hydrolized (broken down) at high degrees. NAN HA contains milk protein and is not suitable for those with cow's milk allergy. It should be taken into consideration that numerous substances to be substituted for milk are not totally valuable in calcium content [22].

In older children, the soy beverage rich in calcium or oat beverage that can be bought in the markets are the suitable ones to be substituted for milk. Rice drink is less valuable in terms of nutritional value. There are a number of soy, oat, rice or palm oil-based products thay can substitute for cream, cheese, yoghurt, ice cream, butter, etc., which provide practical solutions in cooking; yet, their nutritional values vary. Other foods of animal origin, such as meat, poultry, fish and eggs, can usually provide the protein of high value obtained from milk [22].

Lactose intolerance means that purchasing rich products with milk sugar content is limited, which are particularly the curdled milk-based products, ice cream, sweet milk, cream and fresh cheese. The normal cheddar, butter, milk with low lactose content/lactose-free milk and yoghurt contain very little amount of lactose and can be normally used [22].

Other fermented products like kephir/kefir, Biola drink and yoghurt contain lactose, however, due to the fact that the milk acid bacteria can break down lactose themselves, they are generally better tolerated than sweet milk. Separately, the lactase can be purchased in the form of liquid and tablets from a pharmacy. These products allow for getting nutrients with rich lactose content on special occasions, such as cream cake and ice cream. Since many dairy products can be used in the lactose intolerance, the calcium supplement is generally not essential [22].

Individuals who are allergic to eggs should exclude eggs (egg of any animal) and foods made with eggs, food with Albumin and Globulin, mayonnaise, macaroni, etc. from their diets [23].

It is of little importance to remove the egg in egg allergy in terms of the nutritional value. However, it may be difficult to bake good cakes and pies in a totally practical way. Increasing the amount of soda and baking powder and adding cornflour for the colour would usually be sufficient to solve this problem [22].

Fish allergy may be the severe form of food allergy. Whereas those with fish allergy react to any type of fish, some others may react to codfish while tolerating salmon, trout or mackerel [22]. Even some with fish allergy react to the steam that emerges while boiling fish [23]. Those with fish allergy usually tolerate the fish oil owing to the fact that it is purified in terms of proteins. Fish oil is recommended for those with fish allergy because it contains long-chain omega-3 fatty acids, Vitamin D and herb. Seal oil and krill oil can be alternatives to very few of those who react to fish oil. Vitamin D should be taken in as a supplement. The use of dairy products preserves the need for iodine. Numerous ready-made products contain fish in terms of ingredients. As in all the other types of allergies, the descriptions and warnings of the products should be controlled and read with great care [22].

Individuals who are sensitive to fish and seafood may also show allergic reactions to the glues made of the skin of the fish and made of fishbone as well as to the fish and seafood. The glue is a strong allergen and is capable of causing sudden clinic symptoms [23].

Shrimps, crab, crawfish, lobster and other shellfish may lead to allergic and non-allergic reactions. In general, even the little amounts through foods or vapour/steam are enough to cause serious reactions. Since the basic allergen within shellfish are also found in mollusca, such as snail, calamaris (squid) and clams (mussels), the cross reactions among distinct species are common [22,23].

Legume Allergy: Peas, soy beans, lupin flour and peanut belong to the same plant family. Thus, cross reactions may occur among these species. For instance, lupin flour may cause an allergic reaction in some of those allergic to peanuts. Lupin flour is added into several well-cooked or medium-cooked pastery/pie products. Although peanut is found among the products triggering serious allergic reactions, it does not mean that all of those with peanut allergy will suffer from severe reactions. Reacting to the peanut is possible after the intake, or through hand contact or in powder/granulated form [22]. Most of those with peanut allergy may tolerate other tree nuts, it is important to take into consideration that these are usually seen together with food products [23]. Many people prove to be positive to soy in the allergy tests. The reason for this is that soy can cause a cross reaction along with the grass pollen and other legumes. Therefore, it should be guaranteed that soy yields clinical symptoms before excluding it from the nutrient/food [22].

In soy allergy, soy protein must be avoided. However, soy oil and soy lecithin can be used by many since they are based on oil fraction of soy beans. The products labelled as containing vegetable fat do not contain soy protein unless declared in particular [22].

Among the tree nuts are hazelnut, walnut, cashews, pistachio, almond and Brasilian chestnut. One may react to one or more types of nuts [22].

Sesame seed, sunflower seed and poppy seed are the examples of the seeds that may cause allergic reactions. Nut and seed allergy may lead to severe reactions. Hazelnut/nut is found in a number of food products and powder. The reaction is usually seen within a few minutes. For this reason, it is of great significance to read the product description very carefully [22].

Several products are labelled as "it may contain nut marks/traces". They can be consumed but must be very carefully consumed by those who underwent anaphylactic reactions before. The most sensitive ones should avoid nuts or fats/oils produced from seeds, since cold pressed fats may contain a considerable amount of protein residuals. However, those with nut allergy may tolerate oils. Many people show reactions against nuts and almonds only as a cross reaction against the birch tree pollens. Such cross reactions generally indicate slight symptoms and these can usually be tolerated when the nut has been exposed to heat treatment [22].

In wheat allergy; wheat, rye and one or more proteins within barley may trigger allergic symptoms. The positive allergy tests are usually performed for wheat, regardless of any food allergy caused by the intake of wheat. Thus, it is important to verify whether or not there is a clinical allergy, or for instance, whether it is a positive test result due to a grass pollen allergy. When some inhale flour, they may have wheat allergy, but they may also tolerate well by eating foods in which wheat is used as a substance [22].

Corn has less allergen characteristics when compared with the wheat, and for this reason, it is preferred more than wheat. Wheat, on the other hand, is hard to exclude from diets because of its important place in almost any diet. In fact, this situation is also true for the corn. The alpha-amylase trypsin inhibitor is a glycoprotein existing in wheat and is an important allergen type. The food and food elements that should be avoided by the individuals who are allergic to wheat are; bran, crumbs, bulgur wheat, cereal extract, couscous, crackers, durum wheat and durum flour, gluten, macaroni, noodle, malt, soy sauce, starch [23].

Celiac disease, different from the IgE-mediated rapid allergy, involve an immunological reaction to wheat, rye ands barley proteins. In the patients with Celiac disease, the gluten within the food/nutrient, the flattening of the intestines and an inflammation caused by the insufficient intake of nutrients will trigger a reaction. In both cases, the only treatment would be to completely eliminate wheat, barley, rye, spelt, rye wheat, corn wheat, soiled oat and all the products resistant to them [22].

In Celiac disease, the gluten-free diet must definitely be followed-up throughout lifetime. The elimination in wheat protein allergy is preserved singly as long as there is an allergy. When you eliminate the cereals containing gluten, the significant sources for fibres, Vitamin B and trace substances are lost, as well. That is why, today the gluten-free cereals in the supermarkets are recommended for use. The gluten-free oat, corn, buckwheat and seeds are particularly the nutritious alternatives [22].

Fruit and vegetable allergies are generally the cause of cross allergy. As the cross allergy proteins resemble each other, it means that the body does not experience any difference between the substances it is usually allergic to and the proteins within other foods/nutrients. In general, this ailment is perceived as itching and swelling in the mouth, nose, lips and throat. (oral allergy syndrome). This is an irritating situation, yet it is rarely dangerous. In the meantime, symptoms in the stomach, intestines and on the skin occur, as well. Those with birch tree allergy have sense of itching in their mouth when, for instance, a raw carrot or an apple is eaten. However, more often than not, they may still tolerate boiled, fried or canned fruit and vegetables well, whereas some may sense that they react to fruit/vegetables only during the pollen season [22].

In mite allergy, cross reactions may sometimes take place with shellfish and mollusca [22].

In latex allergy, one may experience cross reactions with kiwi, avocado and banana. In grass pollen allergy, the allergy tests generally yield positive results on wheat and legumes; however, this is rarely related with the allergic symptoms [22].

15. Fruit intolerance in the case of eczema

Some fruits may cause irritation on the skin in people with atopic eczema. These are usually histamine-releasing nutrients, such as citrus fruits, strawberries, tomatoes, pineapples and nuts. Separately, chocolate, pork meat, spices and benzoic acid may have such an impact [22].

16. Chocolate

This allergen is important because especially children consume it much, and for this reason it is responsible for the allergic nasal draining, migraine, efflorescence, pruritus, swelling and digestive system disorders. Certain symptoms may appear due to the consumption of chocolate or cacao from the same source [23].

17. Nutrition with the elimination of fruits & vegetables

If we eliminate a number of various fruits and vegetables from our diet, it may mean that the intake of Vitamin C, antioxidants and fibres may be low. Thus, it is important to find out other alternatives to falling in this group of foods to be tolerated. According to several experiences, the fruits like strawberry, raspberry, redcurrant, rosehip and cranberry are well-tolerated by both the children with eczema and those with pollen allergy. Papaya, mango, turnip, various types of cabbages and potatoes are the other examples to the reliable and good sources for Vitamin C and the antioxidants. In addition, there are also strawberry and fruit essence-based nutritional supplements and similar fruit juices [22].

18. Purchasing and Cooking

Read the product description carefully

In food allergy, it is important to read very carefully the list of ingredients / content list of the food products in order to make sure that there is no allergen in question. The manufacturer may sometimes change the food content without any package change, therefore, the description on the label must always be checked. According to the legal notice regulations, the following food allergens shall always be indicated with a mark on the list of ingredients, no matter how small amounts they might have. These are as follows: Gluten-based cereals, milk, shellfish, mollusca, fish, nuts, peanut, celery, mustard, sesame, soy, sesame seed, lupin and sulphur dioxide/sulphide [22].

19. Marking the "...traces..."

Furthermore, several products are marked as " it may contain nuts or " elements of similar traces..". Such a product, as a substance, is manufactured in a machine processing products of a company or also a company processing nuts, however, no nut is added, not even in small amounts [22].

Thus, there may be the risk of nut contamination. Yet, the products marked in this way are safe for many of those with allergies. Only in really serious/severe reactions must such a marking be taken into consideration [22].

20. E-substances

Additives/E-substances are added into the nutrient/food to extend the shelf life or create a texture or colour [22,23]. The additives can be isolated from synthetic manufactured foods or from other foods in a natural way. They are always reported via their own titles or an E-number. The additives never contain milk, lactose, gluten, hazelnut, fish or shellfish [22].

Lyzosyme (E1105) is the sole e-substance that may contain an egg protein. It is not normal to show an allergic reaction to additives. Some colouring agents and preservatives, particularly the benzoic acid components (E210-219) may irritate the current eczema if taken in greater amounts [22].

Individuals with allergy, especially with urticaria and atopic dermatitis, should consume fresh food without additives as much as possible [23].

21. The preparation of foods against food allergy

While cooking, what matters is to prevent any contact of the food being cooked with the nutrient to be avoided as well as making sure that the cutting-boards, ladles and forks, spoons and knives are cleaned well. The kitchen utensils are rinsed after used in cold water, and then they are washed as usual. Cold water helps prevent the proteins from sticking. If some have egg or fish allergy, it may be necessary for them to provide their own cooking pots and pans, while for those with only food allergy, it may be sufficient to provide utensils like ladle, etc. in the preparation of foods [22].

22. Conclusion and recommendations

As it is widely known, food allergy is a situation that affects the human life in an important level. The recent increase in allergic diseases should be considered in detail [5,23].

It is observed that people move away from the traditional food habits in developing and industrializing countries with the changing life styles, and this change is related with the allergy and allergic diseases [23].

Normal birth and feeding with breast milk are important steps foreseen by the nature itself in transferring the microorganisms (friendly bacteria) that manage the health to the babies on the early days of their lives. In the additional nutrients period, food that are rich in friendly bacteria that are presented to us by the nature, and the food that contains fibers that are the food for the friendly bacteria will ensure the continuance of a good health system [18].

People, who prefer the menus that are rich in prebiotic bacteria and their food prebiotics, and who eat natural food in its usual season will live healthier [18].

Author details

Şenay Çetinkaya*

Address all correspondence to: scetinkaya@cu.edu.tr

Pediatric Nursing, Adana School of Health, Çukurova University, Turkey

This subject was presented within the scope of the International Pediatrics Conference at the 11th National Nursing Convention with the participation of the 56th Turkish National Pediatrics Congress and the American Pediatrics Academy (Acapulco Hotel-Girne, Northern Cyprus Turkish Republic Nov. 29th, 2012).

References

[1] Altıntaş D.U. Besin Alerjilerinde Klinik Tablolar ve Tanı. Güncel Pediatri. 2007;3. Ay. 5 (Özel Sayı 1):57-60.

[2] Mısırlıoğlu ED, Bostancı İ. Besin Allerjisi. Türkiye Çocuk Hastalıkları Dergisi (Turkish J Pediatr dis) 2013;4:206-213.

[3] Reading D. The Reality of Food Allergy: The Patients' Perspective. In: Management of Food Allergens. Coutts J, Fielder R. (Edts). Part I Risk Assesment. Blackwell Publishing Ltd. ISBN: 978-1-405-16758-1. 3 Aug 2009. pp. 3-25.

[4] Soyer Ö.U., Adalıoğlu G. Besin Allerjileri. Güncel Çocuk Sağlığı 2007;1(2):204-215.

[5] Sicherer SH. Epidemiology of food allergy. J Allergy Clin Immunol March 2011;127:594-602.

[6] Fiocchi A, Martelli A. Dietary Management of Food Allergy. Pediatric Annals. October 2006;35(10):755-763.

[7] Branum AM, Lukacs SL. Food allergy among children in the United States. Pediatrics 2009;124:1549-1555.

[8] Lack G. Epidemiologic risks for food allergy. J Allergy Clin Immunol 2008;121(6): 1331-1336.

[9] Rona RJ, Keil T, Summers C, Gislason D, Zuidmeer L, Sodergren E, Sigurdardottir ST, Lindner T, Goldhahn K, Dahlstrom J, McBride D, Madsen C. The prevalence of food allergy: A meta-analysis. J Allergy Clin Immunol 2007;120(3): 638-646.

[10] Weiss C, Mun˜oz-Furlong A, Furlong TJ, Arbit J. Impact of Food Allergies on School Nursing Practice. The Journal of School Nursing October 2004; 20(5): 268-278.

[11] Özkan T, Erdemir G. Besin Allerjileri. Güncel Pediatri. 2006;3:75-79.

[12] Ozdemir O, Mete E, Catal F, Ozol D. Food intolerances and Eosinophilic Esophagitis in childhood. Dig Dis Sci 2009;54:8-14.

[13] Sampson HA. Update on food allergy. J Allergy Clin Immunol. 2004 May;113(5): 805-819.

[14] http://www.aid.org.tr/joomla/index.php/hasta-bilgilendirme/allerjik-hastalklar/26-besin-allerjisi/139-besin-alerjilerinin-belirtileri-nelerdir.html Erişim Tarihi: 24.11.2012.

[15] Kim J.S. Food Allergy: Diagnosis, Treatment, Prognosis, and Prevention. Pediatric Annals. August 2008;37(8):546-551.

[16] Somers L. Food allergy: Nutritional considerations for primary care providers. Pediatric Annals. August 2008;37(8):559-568.

[17] Cengizlier R. Besin alerjisi olan süt çocuğuna yaklaşım. Güncel Pediatri. 2007;3. Ay. 5 (Özel Sayı 1):61-63.

[18] Yağcı RV. Probiyotikler ve prebiyotikler niçin önemlidir? ANKEM Derg 2013;27(Ek 2):102-105.

[19] Özdemir Ö. Various effects of different probiotic strains in allergic disorders: an update from laboratory and clinical data. Clin Exp Immunol. 2010 Jun;160(3):295-304.

[20] Galloway, M. Recognising signs of potential food allergy in children. Practice Nurse (PRACT NURSE), Feb 24 2012; 42(3): 26-9.

[21] Galloway, M. Allergy in Child. Practice Nurse; Apr 13 2012; 42 (6):27-30.

[22] Halvorsen R, Landaas VØ, GrØttum HS. Tyrkisk Gıda Allerjisi Araştırma ve Tedavi. Astma-Og Allergoforbundet, Astım ve Allerji Derneği. 2010:1-28 https://www.yumpu.com/tr/document/view/13839186/gda-alerjisi. Erişim Tarihi: 25.07.2014.

[23] Öztürk M, Besler HT. Besin Allerjileri. 2. Baskı. Sağlık Bakanlığı Yayın No: 727, ISBN : 978-975-590-243-2, Ankara: Reklam Kurdu Ajansı Ltd. Şti. 2012: 14-23.

Chapter 3

Child Nonintentional Injury Prevention

Luiz Antonio Del Ciampo and
Ieda Regina Lopes Del Ciampo

Additional information is available at the end of the chapter

http://dx.doi.org/10.5772/58944

1. Introduction

Childhood nonintentional injuries continue to be an important public health problem the world over, involving individuals of different ages and socioeconomic conditions. If, on the one hand, medicine advances in the early detection of diseases, specialized treatments and advanced rehabilitation techniques, on the other, it can be seen that injury continue to an important and relatively little studied cause of morbidity, permanent disability (neurological deficits, amputations, scars, and emotional damage) and death, especially among children [1, 2].

Epidemiological information about childhood injury is still partial and incomplete since this is a multidisciplinary, undefined and very extensive work field that requires the action of qualified and experienced professionals in order to understand the multiple aspects associated with the occurrence of this problem. In addition to obtaining statistical information about mortality and more serious injury, it is necessary to explore the large number of events that remain hidden in the community, with no records in medical care services but very important for the various strategies to be directed at the promotion of health and at the prevention of harm to children's health [30, 39].

2. Epidemiology

More than 2000 children die every day worldwide due to unintentional injury, and many other thousands suffer sequelae and definitive disabilities. According to the World Health Organization, about 10% of the world population is affected by some type of sequelae due to injury, with most of these individuals still being of full reproductive age [14, 27].

In the US, more than 12 million children receive medical care every year due to injury, with more than 132,000 hospital admissions. The annual economic burden is estimated at more than $ 80 billion in medical costs, lost work productivity, lost wages and other expenses [18, 32].

3. Definition

Injury is defined as "an amount of energy (thermal, mechanical, chemical, etc) that exceeds the tolerance capability of the human body and results in damage or lack of vital elements such as oxygen". It is an event independent of the human will provoked by an external force that acts rapidly on an individual and manifests as body and/or mental damage [3, 4].

As is the case for all other diseases, the study of unintentional injury can use the epidemiological model characterized by: a) agent (energy), b) host (child), and c) environment. Thus, injury results from an unfavorable interaction between an etiological agent and a susceptible host, occurring in a determined environment and at a defined moment. On this basis, injuries are not distributed at random among populations, where the interaction between these factors determines the probability and the nature of the event, also considering that the facts accompanying the event are as important as the injury itself [5, 6].

4. The child as a host

The predisposition of children to unintentional injury is related to a large number of socioeconomic, educational and cultural factors. Low income, low educational level of the family, dysfunctionality, difficult access to health services, the use of alcohol and drugs, inadequate supervision, the lack of leisure areas, and unbecoming environments are elements known to be directly related to childhood injury [15, 21, 25].

Regarding children, we should consider their own characteristics which make them more prone to unintentional injury. Thus, within the context of their different developmental stages, we should emphasize physical and emotional immaturity, their inability to anticipate and avoid dangerous situations, their imperfect control of impulses and emotion, great curiosity, inexperience, motivation to perform tasks, tendency to imitate and repeat behaviors, lack of preoccupation about their body, impatience, and limited motor coordination. Also their anatomical peculiarities should be considered, such as skull-body disproportion, the small dimensions of their upper airways, hand-to-mouth personality development, relative weak musculature, large subarachnoid space, cranial bones not fused at the level of the cranial sutures, immature brain, and thin skull. In many situations, children usually must adapt to the world of adults, which is hostile and unknown to them, often having to acquire knowledge by the trial and error method [38].

http://dx.doi.org/10.5772/58944

Epidemiological studies can identify characteristics that help with the construction of the profile of children who are more injury prone. This knowledge is fundamental for the implantation of preventive and educational actions. The main characteristics of this profile are listed below [28, 31].

1. male sex: boys carry out more extroverted and vigorous activities less controlled by adults, with more social requirements and therefore a greater exposure to risks.
2. age of more than one year: the child is able to move by itself, crawling or walking and running, thus expanding its social space and escaping the surveillance of adults.
3. older parents: temporal distance between generations is a factor that complicates the care devoted to the safety and education of the children.
4. large family: when other children share the same physical space, dividing the attention of adults, or when younger children are cared for by other children.
5. physical and/or mental fatigue: children with many social requirements may show physical or emotional stress that makes them more prone to injury due to lack of attention
6. organic or emotional diseases: any factors that may change the dynamic equilibrium of a child are directly related to the occurrence of unintentional injuries at all ages.

5. Age range and types of injuries

Children start from a state of complete physical and mental immaturity and progressively acquire knowledge and skills that permit them to incorporate attitudes of protection and comfort. Thus, and in a more didactic manner, it is possible to point out their main characteristics according to the phase of neuropsychomotor development and the unintentional injuries more commonly occurring in this age range [7, 8, 13, 17, 22].

a. Newborn to 6 months: the infant is completely dependent on adults for its survival (feeding, being kept warm, hygiene, transportation, safety etc.), is immature and unable to control impulses and emotions, thus being prone to some types of injuries such as intoxication with medications, drowning in the bath water, asphyxia with milk, talcum or small objects, scalding with the bath water and feeding bottle, cigarette burns or burns due to prolonged exposure to the sun, traumas in general, especially falling off the carriage, the lap of an adult and during the bath.

b. 7 months to 2 years: the child is acquiring greater voluntary ability to move (rolling in bed, sitting, crawling, walking) and starts the oral phase of personality development, feeling more stimulated by the environment. Starting from this age, any type of injury may occur, the most common being falls, burns, intoxications, suffocation, ingestion of foreign bodies, being run over, aggression by venomous animals, animal bites, drowning, and electric shock.

c. up to 2 years of age, the neuromotor development of the child becomes more specialized, the child expands its social environment and is less dependent on adults, who also, naturally, start reducing their surveillance of the child. They have great curiosity, a low ability to anticipate risks, they are unaware of danger and they imitate various behaviors, thus being exposed to a large number of risks such as being run over, drowning, falls, burns, intoxications, electrical shocks, animal bites, and aggression by venomous animals. After five years of age, children are more developed, with a greater ability to learn and to protect themselves, but they still suffer external influences and are little supervised by adults, continuing to be exposed to the same risks.

Practically half the unintentional injuries in the whole world occur at home, i.e., in the place where children spend most of their time. In the domestic environment, the sites of higher risk are: a) the kitchen, which contains sharp or pointed objects, a stove, gas, appliances and cleaning products; b) the backyard/garden, where leisure activities and sports practice occur and where pets are raised, and/or which serve as work areas for the family; c) the room where the family gathers for the meals, for evening leisure and for receiving visits. Thus, the domestic environment, either because of its poverty or because of its increasing sophistication due to technological development, becomes highly dangerous for children, since the progress of comfort for human beings is not always accompanied by the necessary safety measures. Outside the home, the street and the school greatly contribute to the high rates of injuries predominating among children older than five years.

6. Characteristics of unintentional injuries

Seasonality is also related to the occurrence of injuries, with a higher incidence of these events on weekends or during school vacation (especially the European and North American summer), when the warmer and more agreeable climate stimulates physical and leisure activities, competitions, trips etc. During the winter, when people spend more time at home and in closed environments, other types of unintentional injuries can also occur, especially intoxication due to alcoholic drinks [12, 29].

7. Prevention

Unintentional injuries are an endemic problem that requires permanent actions for its prevention and/or control. The predisposition of children can only be neutralized by the adults responsible for their education and safety. In this respect, the identification of risk factors is necessary in order to elaborate Prevention and Control Programs, which should contemplate strategies at the primary level such as prevention of new injuries; strategies at the secondary level such as reduction of injury severity, and strategies at the tertiary level such as reduction of the frequency and severity of the sequelae [33-37].

According to the classical Haddon Injury Control Model, injuries are due to energy (thermal, chemical, kinetic, radiation and electric) that is transferred to the child by a determined vector.

http://dx.doi.org/10.5772/58944

Thus, measures aiming at avoiding or reducing the effects of this energy transfer should be implemented in order to protect the individuals [19, 20].

The main measures that can be adopted are:

a. avoiding the release of energy

b. distancing the individual from the source of energy

c. reducing the quantity of released energy

d. using barriers between energy and the body

e. strengthening the structure that receives energy

f. modifying the surface of contact

g. modifying the space distribution of energy

Thus, efforts should be directed at expanded health education actions according to each social reality, involving health services appropriate for care that will reduce sequelae, family and social rehabilitation and reintegration, the training of professionals of all categories that deal with children, and appropriate legislation directed at the prevention of unintentional injuries and at the protection of vulnerable persons. Communication among citizen, public health researchers and legislators are necessary to promote more effective policymaking. Anticipatory guidance in pediatric practice, to children, parents and society as a whole, expanding the educational level can improve general safety behaviors.

It should be pointed out that prevention involves education, instruction and advocating for changes to improve child safety, such as changes in the environment and in various products, and the elaboration and application of laws aiming at the protection of children. Physicians and all other health professionals who are aware of the peculiarities of children, of the family environment and of habits and attitudes should practice preventive medicine. All they need for this purpose is to incorporate the basic principles of home safety and injury prevention into their habitual conduct, transmitting them in the form of guidance and counseling during medical visits, home visits or group meetings of parents and caregivers. It is possible to establish differentiated guidelines for each age range based on the stage of neuropsychomotor development and on the awareness of the social reality in which the child is inserted, always using common sense and logic as the framework for the establishment of a safe and healthy environment for the child.

With the effort and participation of the entire community, especially of its leaders and of its more differentiated segments, decisively acting in order to be able to modify environments and/or behaviors, it will be possible to correct the more critical situations and to mitigate the damage caused by unintentional injuries to children's health [9-11,16,23-26].

Anticipatory Guidance for Injury Prevention

Always supervise the child's activities

Newborn to 6 months

- breastfeed the child in a sitting position
- child should sleep supine
- avoid using pillows
- remove loose bedding clothes, quilts, stuffed toys and soft objects from cradle
- check temperature of bath water
- avoid prolonged sun exposure
- do not use talc
- do not use drugs without medical advice
- avoid toys with sharp objects, sharp edges, loose paint or disassemble it into small pieces
- bed should have protective grilles
- do not handle hot liquids or food with child in lap
- do not leave the baby in the care of another child

7 months to 2 years

- do not leave medicines, herbs or small objects within reach of children; store in a safe place
- use of protective electrical outlets
- do not leave child unattended while bathing near the pool, river, beach, pond, or large containers with water
- do not leave your child unattended at sites that are uneven or near windows
- use gates for starways and pool fencing
- use protective grilles on windows, pools, stairs and elevated parts of the house
- hinder children's access to home appliances
- keep combustible chemicals, cleaning materials and liquids out of the reach of children
- keep sheets and blankets always stuck to the mattress
- avoid contact of the child with candy, food into small pieces and fruit pits
- beware of ornamental plants,
- keep plastic packaging, ribbons and cords out of the reach of children
- avoid contact with animals, whether domestic, which should always be healthy and vaccinated,
- use appropriate equipment (child restraints) for transporting children in vehicles
- do not use infant walkers

Up to 2 years

- beware of high places, furniture that can be scaled and unstable objects of decoration
- do not leave your child alone in the kitchen or service area of the house
- keep sharp objects, knives and tools out of the reach of children
- do not leave children unattended in streets, parks, places with a lot of movement of people and vehicles
- store medicines in a safe place
- do not use food packaging to keep harmful products to health
- always keep clean the yards, gardens and grounds adjacent to the house
- keep tubs, tanks and buckets empty after use
- avoid handling of fireworks
- cycling with helmet, elbow and knees pads, and appropriate locations
- installing energy-absorbing surfacing material in playgrounds
- teach basic rules of conduct in traffic, because the child is passing pedestrian and vehicle

http://dx.doi.org/10.5772/58944

Author details

Luiz Antonio Del Ciampo * and Ieda Regina Lopes Del Ciampo

*Address all correspondence to: delciamp@fmrp.usp.br

Add affiliations, Country

References

[1] Along O, Hyder AA. Reducing the global burden of childhood unintentional injuries. Arch Dis Child 2014;99:62-9.

[2] Baker S, O'Neill B, Guinsburg MJ, Li G. Baker SP. The injury fact book, 2nd ed. Lexington, MA, Lexington Books, 1992.

[3] Bell N, Schuurman N. GIS and injury prevention and control: history, challenges and opportunities. Int J Environ Res Public Health 2010;7:1002-7.

[4] Bourdillon M. Children in development. Progress in Development Studies 2004;4:99-113.

[5] Brussoni M, Towner E, Hayes M. Evidence into practice: combining at the art and science on injury prevention. Injury Prevention 2006;12:373-7.

[6] Centers for Disease Control and Prevention. National Center for Injury Prevention and Control. National action plan for child injury prevention. An agenda to prevent injuries and promote the safety of children and adolescents in the United States. http://www.cdc.gov/safechild/pdf/National_Action_Plan_for_Child_Injury_Prevention.pdf.

[7] Collins NC, Molcho M, Carney P, McEvoy L, Geoghegan L, Phillips JP et al. Are boys and girls that different? An analysis of traumatic brain injury in children. Emerg Med J 2013;30:675-8.

[8] Del Ciampo LA, Ricco RG. Acidentes na Infância. Pediatria, S. Paulo 1996;18:193-197.

[9] Del Ciampo LA, Ricco RG, Muccillo G. Acidentes domésticos na infância na área de Vila Lobato, Ribeirão Preto-SP. Pediatria (S.Paulo) 1997;19:38-42.

[10] Del Ciampo LA, Ricco RG, Muccillo G. Acidentes: sabemos preveni-los? Pediatria (S. Paulo) 1997;19:263-266.

[11] Fang X, Jing R, Zeng G, Linnan HW, Zhu X, Linnan M. Socioeconomic status and the incidence of child injuries in China. Social Science & Medicine 2014;102:33-40.

[12] Gracey M. Child health in an urbanizing world. Acta Paediatrica 2002;91:1-8.

[13] Grossman DC. The history of injury control and the epidemiology of child and adolescent injuries. The Future of Children 2000;10:23-52

[14] Haddon W Jr. On the escape of tigers: an ecologic note. American Journal of Public Health and the Nation's Health 1970; 60:2229-34.

[15] Haddon W Jr. Energy damage and the ten countermeasure strategies. Journal of Trauma 1973;13:321-31.

[16] Imamura JH, Troster EJ, Oliveira CAC. What types of unintentional injuries kill our children? Do infants die of the same types of injuries? A systematic review. Clinics 2012;67:1107-16.

[17] Jones G, Steketee RW, Black RE, Bhutta ZA, Morris SS. How many child deaths can we prevent this year? Lancet 2003;362:65-71.

[18] Kendrick D, Mulvaney CA, Ye L, Stevens T, Mytton JA, Stewart-Brown S. Parenting interventions for the prevention of unintentional injuries in childhood. Cochrane Database Syst Rev. 2013 Mar 28;3:CD006020. doi: 10.1002/14651858.CD006020.pub3.

[19] Krug EG. Injury surveillance is key to preventing injuries. Lancet 2004:364:1563-6.

[20] Liyanage IK, Pathirana AC, Wickramasinghe KK, Karunathilake IM, Olupaliyawa A. A study of risk factors for non-intentional domestic injuries among preschoolers in three suburban areas of Sri Lanka. Asia Pac J Pub Health 2008;20:156-61.

[21] Luckhoff C, Starr C. Minor head injuries in children. Australian Family Physician 2010;39:284-8

[22] Lyons RA. Modification of the home environment for reduction of injuries. Cochrane Database of Systematic Reviews 2003,4:CD003600.

[23] Majsak-Newman G, Benford P, Ablewhite J, Clacy R, Coffey F, Cooper N. et al. Keeping children safe at home: protocol for a matched case control-study of modifiable risk factors for poisoning. Injury Prevention 2014; Apr 7. doi: 10.1136/injuryprev-2014-041234

[24] Marsac ML, Donlon K, Berkowitz S. Indicated and selective preventive interventions. Child and Adolescent Psychiatric Clinics of North America 2014;23:383-97.

[25] Melzer-Lange MD, Zonfrillo MR, Gittelman MA. Injury Prevention. Opportunities in the Emergency Department. Pediatric Clinics of North America 2013;60:1241-53.

[26] Miller TR, Romano EO, Spicer RS. The cost of childhood unintentional injuries and the value of prevention. Future Child 2000;10:137-63.

[27] Miller SM. Injury prevention and control: reflections on the state and direction of the field. Sal Pub Mex 2008;50:101-11.

[28] Mock C, Quansah R, Krishnan R, Arreola-Risa C, Rivara F. Strengthening the prevention and care of injuries worldwide. Lancet 2004;363:2172-9.

[29] Norton R, Kobusingye O. Injuries. New England Journal of Medicine 2013;368:1723-30.

[30] Olawoye OA, Iyun AO, Adenola SA, Michael AI, Oluwatosin OM. Demographic characteristics and prognostic indicators of childhood burn in a developing countries. Burns 2014;jun 2 (epub ahead of print).

[31] Pronczuk J, Surdu S. Children's environmental health in the twenty-first century. Annals of New York Academy Sciences 2008;1140:143-54.

[32] Smithson J, Garside R, Pearson M. Barriers to, and facilitators of, the prevention of unintentional injury in children in the home:a systematic review and synthesis of qualitative research. Inj Prev 2011;17:119-26.

[33] Sutchritpongsa S, Sangwisit S, Sonjaipanich S. Parental awareness of household injury prevention: adequacy of anticipatory guidance for well childcare. Journal of Medical Association of Thailand. 2013;96:1531-5.

[34] Theurer WM, Bhavsar AK. Prevention of unintentional childhood injury. American Family Physician 2013;87:502-9.

[35] Towner E, Towner J. The prevention of childhood unintentional injury. Current Paediatrics 2001;11:403-8.

[36] Towner E, Dowswell T. Community-based childhood injury prevention: what works? Health Promotion International 2002;17:273-84.

[37] Weber P, Jenni O. Screening in child health. Deutsches Arzteblatt International 2012;109:431-5.

[38] WHO. World Report on Child Injury Prevention. Switzerland, 2008.

Chapter 4

Osteomyelitis and Nursing Management

Şenay Çetinkaya and Sibel Kuşdemir

Additional information is available at the end of the chapter

http://dx.doi.org/10.5772/59142

1. Introduction

Osteomyelitis can be described as the inflammation of bone and bone marrow and it usually indicates the presence of an infection. Although the term of osteomyelitis among children usually expresses acute hematogenous osteomyelitis, it may occur as sub-acute and rarely as chronic. Although bacteria are the main cause for it, fungi, parasites and other microorganisms can also be responsible [1-3].

2. General facts

2.1. Epidemiology

The incidence of osteomyelitis in the first two decades is the highest. 50% of the cases occur among children under the age of 5. The rate of occurrence among patients with sickle cell anemia and people whose immune system is suppressed is high [4]. Except for the first year of life, the male female incidence rate is 2:1. Prior to the infection among 1/3 of the patients, a minor trauma history is found. Genetic and socio-economic factors are also influential in the process of formation of the disease [2,3].

2.2. Pathogenesis and pathology

Osteomyelitis cases among children may occur hematogenously, and more likely the metaphysis of the long bones are involved (especially the distal femur, proximal tibia) [5,6].

Microorganisms may infect bones in three ways:

a. Direct inoculation (trauma, during surgical operation).

b. From an infection in a nearby area (like cellulitis), local invasion [7,8].

c. Hematogenously spreading out (bacterial) is the most common case.

The reason for this is that the capillaries in the metaphysis area show a sinus-like expansion, besides that the endothelial cells that are located around the ven area in the arterioles of the metaphysis lack the ability of phagocytosis. The capillaries in the metaphysis pose a suitable area for the location of microorganisms because the blood current here is low and it is a suitable nourishing place, on the other hand the state that around the capillary veins there are no phagocytic cells may result in a vulnerable environment [4, 9]. As a result, bacteria that come through the blood stream may easily multiply in the metaphysis sinusoids and the sinusoids will become filled with pus and form an abscess. Because of the ischemia caused by the abscess in the medullary bone necrosis will start. As the volume of the abscess increases, so does the intramedullary pressure, and cortical ischemia develops in this area. Later the abscess will reach to the sub-periosteal gap via the Haversian system and cause sub-periosteal abscess. "Sequestra" is the name for bone parts whose blood supply are impaired and are separated from living bone parts, and "involucrum" is called for healthy bone parts surrounding the dead bone parts. Meanwhile, new bone formation continues from the endosteal and periosteal. As a result, in the bones 1) inflammation and formation of abscess (with the influence of bacteria and enzymes) 2) necrosis (vascular obstruction) 3) pathological changes due to new bone formation processes will be observed [7].

Among children the effects of osteomyelitis may show difference according to age. Under the age of two, the nutrition of the epiphysis is obtained by the metaphysis veins that intercross the physis. Through these veins, the infection in the metaphysis may pass to the epiphysis. It may even spread to the joint and be the cause to the septic arthritis. Damage to the physis may be cause to separation of the epiphysis, deformities and extremity shortness. Diaphyseal involvement is rare except very heavy cases. Above two years of age, by taking role as a barrier, the physis borders the metaphysis from the infection, and prevents it from spreading to the epiphysis and the joint cavity. After the closing of the physis, the infection may spread from the metaphysis to the epiphysis, and it may form septic arthritis [2,7,10].

If the infection is not treated in the acute period, chronic osteomyelitis is unavoidable. Then, the surrounding of the infection-focus filled with pus and granulation tissue will be surrounded by a fibrous capsule and sclerosing bone-tissue and the "Brodie" abscess will be formed [9].

2.3. Etiology

The main cause among children at all ages is the *Staphylococcus aureus.* In a lower rate *Group A, streptococci* and *Streptococcus pneumoniae* may be observed. *Haemophilus influenza* and *Gram negative enteric bacteria* are becoming increasingly important in the etiology of osteomyelitis in areas where routine vaccination isn′t practiced in the first year of life. In the newborn period (0-4 weeks) Group B streptococci, Escherichia coli (E. coli) and gram-negative bacteria are the major microorganisms that cause osteomyelitis. In penetrating injuries and IV drug addicts *Pseudomonas auruginosa,* in sickle cell anemia *Salmonella strain,* in chronic hemodialysis patients *coagulase-negative staphylococci* and *S. aureus,* and in chronic granulomatous disease *Serratia* and *Spergillus strains* are the expected pathogens. Fungal osteomyelitis especially occurs among newborns, immune-suppressed patients and intravenous drug users [3]. Tuberculosis osteomyelitis in less developed countries still constitutes the main cause of musculoskeletal infections. *Mycobacterium tuberculosis* most frequently grips the vertebral body and the synovial. In recent years, without primary lung focus osteomyelitis patients with single focused tuberculosis osteomyelitis have been reported. Although rare, tuberculosis osteomyelitis may develop due to tuberculosis vaccine (Bacillus-Calmette-Guerin; BCG vaccine). Among approximately half of the children with acute osteomyelitis, a bacterial etiology cannot be detected. *Staphylococcus aureus* and *gram-negative enterics* are the most common causes of chronic osteomyelitis. From pathogenic microorganisms, usually furuncles, impetigo, deep or superficial abscess, carious teeth and infected tonsils like primary focuses come to the bone via the blood. Any types of trauma that cause to bacteremia are important risk factors in the formation of the disease [9].

2.4. Clinical table

In osteomyelitis, clinical findings vary according to age. Because babies possess a weaker anatomic barrier to limit the spreading of infections among them, they show a tendency for the disease; and together with it, the septic arthritis, soft tissue infection and pseudo-paralysis of the affected extremity are widespread. Among older children, the infection is more focal. Most frequently, there is fever and ache at the infection location. More rarely, there may be loss of appetite, malaise and vomiting. The patient will be reluctant to use the extremity. Depending on the osteomyelitis, deep venous thrombosis may develop and it may be the first consultancy reason [7,10].

2.4.1. Age factor

Newborn Form: Among newborns, findings are very weak, when the affected extremity is touched or moved, the baby becomes disturbed. Around the pseudo-paralysis, there may develop a swelling. The newborn osteomyelitis consists of residual deformities, frequent infections of the multiple bones, and the involvement of the joints, facial bones and the proximal humerus. The onset is often hidden, following umbilical artery catheterization or the taking heel blood swelling or decreased activity may occur. There may be no fever or leukocytosis. Although there is an inclusion of a large number of bacteria species Staphylococcus aureus, Candida albicans and the group B Streptococci are observed as the most common pathogens [10].

Bone scans can detect clinically undefined points. Any joint affected is drained immediately. In newborns, usually in the bone cortex, a window-like drilling surgery is not necessary [10].

Baby form: it occurs among patients younger than the age of 1, and it often spreads from the epiphysis to the metaphysis and joints while the veins of the diaphysis enter into the epiphysis. The periosteum often becomes rapidly perforated and it becomes rapidly pierced. The cover (new bone development belonging to one periosteum) formation may be large but due to absorption and reformation, it is temporary. If it inhibits a long bone, with the shortening of the organ, the epiphyseal growth centers may become damaged [10].

Childhood Form: This type generally occurs among patients from 1 year of age until puberty. It is usually settled in the metaphysis and doesn′t spread to the epiphysis, as the veins do not enter the epiphyseal plaque. It rarely damages the growth cartilage or the joint [10].

Adult Form: This type reveals after the age of 16. The growth cartilage dissolves and the metaphyseal infection may spread to the epiphysis and the joint. Chronic infection is more common among adults in comparison to children [10].

2.4.2. Specific findings in the bones

Long bones: For long bones, acute hematogenous osteomyelitis is typical. In around 70% of the cases, the femur or tibia are affected. When there is no osteomyelitis area, it is more difficult to diagnose, usually it is in the metaphysis but it occurs in the diaphysis rather more (in the center) or epiphysis (in the center) of the long bone. To diagnose osteomyelitis of the femoral neck is difficult since negative findings in the joint resemble hip arthritis. Besides interruption of blood supply to the femoral head or as a result of the insertion penetration the osteomyelitis in the femoral neck area may be the cause to heavy hip-joint complications [7,10].

Feet: Puncture wounds of the foot, especially those in the metatarsal area may result in soft tissue, bone and particularly of the cartilage *Pseudo aeruginosa* infection. Typically, the patient may possess a wound through shoes and a developing swelling will heal in the first day or afterwards. Often, local pain is an important clue, but fever and leukocytosis in generally is mild or absent. When there is redness or swelling at the toes, a couple of days later, an exploratory surgery with the debridement of the area is nearly always necessary to the foot sole wound. Radiologic evidence of bone destruction generally may not be observed for several weeks. Scanning sometimes helps. The recovery of *Pseudomonas* on aspirated substance culture will yield to the determination of more demand for debridement [10].

Clavicle: Particularly among drug addicts, clavicle or a sternoclavicular joint is sometimes an area where sub-acute infection is built up. Osteomyelitis of the clavicle occurs also among children [10].

Patella: Patella osteomyelitis may be confused with suprapatellar bursitis for it is very seldom [10].

Fingers: Pyogenic osteomyelitis arises in many fingertip abscesses as a complication. Without a neighbor that is infected, the osteomyelitis of a finger bone may lead to a secondary tuberculosis case [10].

Rib: Rib excision will dry the osteomyelitis and secrete the agent to prevent the Ewing's sarcoma or other tumors. Generally, it will be accompanied by chest pain and fever [10].

Pelvis: Pelvic osteomyelitis will include pubis, ilium and ischium. Often, there will be fever, abnormal gait and severe sensitivity in the affected bone area. Roentgenographic changes may last from 10 days to 10 weeks. *Staphylococcus aureus* is the common cause. Bone scans are useful but may be negative in the early stages. Ultrasound may show the displacement of the bladder [10].

Vertebra: Vertebral body infection is rare in children. But, intervertebral disc infection, i.e. discitis is common. Generally, the source can't be found [10].

Other Bones: Cranial osteomyelitis typically is an extension of otitis externa, mastoiditis, or sinusitis. It occurs after multiple antibiotics use and usually causes Pseudomonas aeruginosa [10].

2.5. Diagnosis

Several microbiological, haematological, serological and radiological tests are useful in the clinical diagnosing and the determination of the causative factors of the disease [6]. In an age in which the prevalence of antibiotic-resistant microorganisms is increasing, extreme effort is required to determine the specific etiology of the disease. For directing the anti-microbial treatment, it is imperative to obtain pathogen sensitivity tests. The diagnostic methods described below can be applied to all forms of osteomyelitis [7,9].

2.5.1. Laboratory findings

In osteomyelitis laboratory findings are nonspecific. The erythrocyte sedimentation rate (ESR) is usually measured in the range of 40-60 mm/hr; it reaches the highest rate within 3-5 days of the treatment, and it returns to normal within 3 weeks. As ESR gradually decreases with successful treatment, elevated ESR is a perfect parameter for monitoring the response to the treatment. The rise of the C-reactive protein (CRP) level is the highest on 2nd day of the treatment (mean 83 mg/L) and it drops to normal in 1 week. This, together with the ESR, is used for monitoring response to the treatment [3].

The etiologic diagnosis of osteomyelitis is performed by isolating the microorganism from the bone, sub-periosteal exudate and joint fluid [3].

Blood cultures should be obtained from all patients with possible osteomyelitis. The blood cultures of approximately 50% of the patients with acute hematogenous osteomyelitis are positive. Newborn osteomyelitis is often characterized with bacteremia. As in other osteomyelitis forms, the probability of the blood cultures to be positive is lower in osteomyelitis that is developing from the neighboring focus, like the osteomyelitis that is accompanying chronic osteomyelitis and peripheral vascular disease. In this context, blood culture is a limited guide. A separate set of two or four cultures should be taken [9].

There may be leukocytosis but cases in which the leukocyte number is normal or slightly higher occur often, and therefore it cannot be used to rule out the osteomyelitis diagnosis [9].

2.5.2. *Radiologic findings*

Conventional radiography for diagnosis of pediatric patients is necessary. In osteomyelitis, the usual development sequence of radiographic changes is as follows:

1. In the early stages of the disease, the direct radiographs are normal. At this stage, bone scintigraphy can detect abnormal findings. However, if there is bone destruction, further imaging is not necessary.

2. Stage: 3 days after the onset of symptoms in the metaphyseal area, a localized deep soft tissue swelling is observed. Soft tissue swelling and an increase in the subperiost are the earliest detected abnormalities.

3. After 3 to 7 days of the onset, swelling in the muscles and a deletion in the translucent oil lines is observed.

4. Stage: 10-21 days after the start of the findings of bone destruction, lytic lesions, periosteal removal due to the accumulation of purulent subcortical and periosteal new bone formation becomes apparent. Lytic changes may not be visible in direct graphics until the 30% to 50% of the bone disappears and are not detectable until after 2-6 weeks of the onset of the disease. Sclerotic changes may occur weeks after the onset of the disease after the formation of the new matrix due to a delay in mineralization. Sclerotic changes associated with periosteal new bone formation (involucrum) indicate the presence of a more chronic process [9].

Magnetic Resonance imaging is a suitable method for the examination of the bone, and in comparison to computed tomography, it will better reveal the pus accumulation in subperiosteal and soft tissues. This is the preferred method for the diagnosis of vertebral osteomyelitis. In the diagnosis of acute osteomyelitis, its sensitivity is close to 100% and, in addition to this, it is useful in the differentiation of acute and chronic osteomyelitis. Radionuclide studies are helpful in early stage diagnosis even when there are no findings with plain radiography. However, its use is limited among newborns [7].

In comparison to radiologic examinations, bone scintigraphy is more valuable for osteomyelitis [2,7,9,10]. Among technetium radio-phosphate, scintigraphic methods especially the three-phase are the most used ones. Radiation exposure is approximately the same as the standard radiography and children patients are not contraindicated. Because of referred pain or the probability of a multifocal infection, the whole-body scintigraphy of patients who are suspected to have osteomyelitis should be done. Afterwards, a more thorough detailed radiologic investigation of the suspected areas can be made. Scintigraphy done with indium-labeled leukocytes is an excellent sensitivity and specificity method in the determination of early osteomyelitis. This method is technically a little more difficult, and has more radiation levels when compared with the bone scintigraphies with technetium [9].

Needle aspiration must be practiced to every patient whose absolute diagnosis has not been performed via blood cultures to obtain sample cultures from lesions inside bones, from the collection of soft tissues, from the abscesses under the periosteum. Preferably, needle aspiration should be practiced prior to giving antibiotics. If there is joint effusion together with it, synovial fluid tests should be performed. The aspired effusion should be investigated regarding the cells it contains, and in terms of biochemistry, Gram straining and culture [9].

Patients among whom the exact etiology cannot be determined despite the blood cultures or needle aspiration, especially when tuberculosis, fungal or a malignant disease is suspected, open biopsy may be considered. The biopsy samples should be reserved for histopathological analysis and for cultures that are regarded necessary [7,9].

2.5.3. Differential diagnosis

In cases with possible high fever, pain and sensitivity in the extremities, the differential diagnosis should be performed. Rheumatic fever, septicemia, septic arthritis, cellulitis, Ewing's sarcoma, metastatic neuroblastoma, leukemia, reflex neurovascular dystrophy, to thrombophlebitis hemoglobinopathies connected bone infarcts and toxic synovitis can be counted to be in these cases [2,3].

2.6. Treatment

The initial treatment can be intense. Inadequate treatment of acute osteomyelitis can result in relapse and the development of chronic disease [3,11]. The treatment should be adjusted to the patient's characteristics (Table 1 and 2).

2.6.1. Antibiotics using principles

The basic choice of antibiotics and although the number of comparative studies for the determination of the duration of the treatment is few, antibiotics are the mainstay of the treatment [9].

2.6.1.1. Parenteral antibiotic treatment

Usually in the beginning of the treatment, to be sure of the harmony and to reach the necessary bone levels, parenteral agents are recommended. Because the passage of antibiotics to the bone is low, these agents are generally given in high doses [6]. The passage of antibiotics is linked to the vascularization of the bone (e.g., the surfaces in spongiform bone tissue are higher than in cortical bone). The levels of antibiotics in diseased bone are even higher. Penicillin, cephalosporins, gentamicin, vancomycin, clindamycin and ciprofloxacin reach to a level that exceeds the Minimal Inhibitory Concentration (MIC) of many of the susceptible microorganisms that lead to osteomyelitis [12]. When the obtained serum levels are considered, especially clindamycin and ciprofloxacin pass well into the bone. Indeed, whether you give these agents intravenously or orally, the treatment of them has been proven for all forms of osteomyelitis [2,9].

Patient Characteristics	Possible Pathogen	Antibiotics Selection
Empirical treatment	Staphylococcus aureus Haemophilus influenzae type b	nafcillin/clindamycin/ vancomycin (MRSA*) cefuroxime/cefotaxime/ ceftriaxone/ chloramphenicol
Newborn	S. Aureus Group B streptococcus Gram negative enteric bacteria	nafcillin* cefotaxime/gentamicin
<5 years	S. Aureus Streptococci H. influenza type	nafcillin + Cefotaxime/Ceftriaxone OR Cefuroxime OR Ampicillin-sulbactam
>5 years	Gram positive cocci	Nafcillin OR Clindamycin OR Cefazolin
Sickle cell anemia	S. Aureus Coliform bacteria	Nafcillin/Clindamycin+ Cefotaxime/ Ceftriaxone
Puncture injuries Partially broken	S. Aureus Anaerobe bacteria	Clindamycin
Immunosuppressed patients	MRSA Pseudomonas aeruginasa	Vancomycin + ceftazidime ticarcillin-clavulanate
Puncture foot injury	P. Aeruginasa	Ceftazidime/mezlosilin+ Aminoglycosides AND Surgical Debridement
Remained in the hospital for a long time preterm	MRSA Resistant gram negative bacteria Antifungal agents	Vancomycin Carbapenems Fungus

MRSA* : methicillin-resistant Staphylococcus aureus

Table 1. Treatment approach in acute osteomyelitis [3].

Medicine	Dose (mg/kg/day)	Daily dose
Nafcillin	150	4
Clindamycin	30	3-4
Cephazolin	100	3
Cefotaxime	150	4
Ceftriaxone	100	2
Cefuroxime	150	3
Ampicillin-Sulbactam	300	4
Gentamicin	5-7.5	3

Table 2. Antibiotics doses in acute osteomyelitis [3]

2.6.1.2. Oral antibiotics treatment

Patients will be treated with intravenous antibiotics for 5-10 days. After a good clinical response, the treatment of the patient is changed into a high-dose oral treatment and this continues for at least 3 weeks. One should especially focus on some aspects of the oral treatment.

a. For susceptibility tests, one should obtain an active organism and it should be sensitive to the selected agent. In vitro sensitivity tests help to select the appropriate treatment. As a long-term treatment is necessary in this disease, it is vital that sensitivity tests are performed carefully. Because, combinations of antibiotics may lead to additional toxicity, if sensitivity combinations are not well known, the best way is to stay away from such combinations.

b. Surgical debridement and drainage should be performed in a suitable manner.

c. One should be certain about the harmony. If there is a doubt about the patient's adhering to the treatment, then treating the patient outside the hospital should be avoided.

d. Some professionals defend that the serum bactericidal levels should be used in order to observe the effectiveness of the treatment. In this method, blood is taken from the patient just before and right after giving the antibiotics. Later on, serial dilutions of the serum are analyzed for the bactericidal activity to the active microorganism. But, as there is no standard protocol and there are no large studies to support this test, its real value is not known.

e. The extension of the treatment is very important and the use of the antibiotics should be continued for at least 4-6 weeks. The rate of healing is expected to be more than 90% [9].

Medicine	Dose(mg/kg/day)	Daily dose
Amoxicillin	100	4
Cefaclor	150	4
Cephalexin	100-150	4
Chloramphenicol	75	3
Clindamycin	30-40	3
Cloxacillin	125	4
Dicloxacillin	75-100	4
Penicillin V	125	6

Table 3. Oral antibiotics doses in acute osteomyelitis [3]

2.6.2. Surgical drainage

Nearly all of the hematogenous osteomyelitis will heal without surgery when treated with suitable doses of antibiotics. In the treatment after 3 to 5 days from the beginning of the disease, the results are even better. Yet, these patients should be monitored by an orthopedic surgeon in the future to evaluate a surgical necessity [9].

The surgical indications include the following:

a. Diagnosis: When pathogens are not determined in blood cultures for sure, diagnostic aspiration should be performed routinely.

b. Hip joint involvement (osteomyelitis of femoral metaphysis): In these cases, it is imperative to drain early because of the tearing risk of the cortex and the possibility of the infection to spread into the hip joint.

c. The neurological complications of vertebral or cranial osteomyelitis.

d. Poor response or non-response to the treatment: If patients do not respond well clinically after 48-72 hours of the treatment, drainage operation is necessary. Among patients whose disease has occurred with gram-negative enteric bacilli, drainage is more often a requisite. A collection of pus under the periosteum that does not respond has to be drained too. A culture should be taken from all the surgical samples.

e. Sequestrum: They need to be removed surgically [9].

Even in the case of a suitable antibiotics treatment among children and adolescents with CA-MRSA (Community-associated methicillin-resistant S. Aureus), incision and drainage were found to be necessary in osteomyelitis. Besides, when the child doesn′t respond to the antibiotics treatment, surgical drainage should be considered. In such a case, surgical initiative can enhance the healing. In addition to this, surgical initiative will allow microbiological evaluation of the tissue collection to confirm the diagnosis of histological analysis of unusual causes of osteomyelitis [13].

http://dx.doi.org/10.5772/59142

2.7. Prognosis

The treatment results of children with acute hematogenous osteomyelitis who do not have complications are fine. Together with this, the prognosis is in relation with different factors. These factors include the active organism, the duration of the symptoms before the treatment, age and the duration of the antibiotics treatment [2].

Sufficient antibiotics treatment is essential. Among 10% to 20% of the patients who are treated for acute hematogenous osteomyelitis, recurrence is observed [2].

Among patients who have osteomyelitis due to gram-negative organisms, the recurrence rate is higher [2].

For completely healing, the best opportunity is the initial treatment. Only 50% of recurrent infection patients with full debridement and intravenous antibiotics for 4-6 weeks can heal. To prevent acute osteomyelitis chronic infections, one should be treated in an effective way and in adequate time interval [2,9].

Before the start of antibiotics, acute hematogenous osteomyelitis was a disease with a high morbidity and mortality rate. With the discovery of ways of diagnosis and cure and in a changing world, the mortality rate of the disease have become unimportant. Despite this, for various reasons, the clinical course of children with acute hematogenous osteomyelitis makes it difficult to apply standard treatment recommendations. The treatment should be always individualized with a team approach that include pediatric infection professionals and orthopedists [13].

Without regarding the attainability of all new microbial agents, the major therapeutic concern in all forms of osteomyelitis is to start with the most appropriate treatment as soon as possible. In this context two concepts are important; the first one, the difficulty in certifying the existence at the appropriate time, and the second one is the determination of the alleged pathogen and the opportunity to assess the antibiotics resistance [13].

3. Special forms of osteomyelitis

3.1. Chronic osteomyelitis

The patient was previously treated for osteomyelitis at the same location. The prognosis is worse than acute osteomyelitis. Treatment failure rate is higher than with the acute form and the way of treatment is different [9].

The patient rarely shows acute symptoms. Systemic symptoms like fever are not common. Except for drainage from the sinus or the wound, regional signs and findings are less common [2].

Among the causes, *Staphylococcus aureus* is the most common pathogen. *Staphylococcal* infections can recur after many years the initial episode. Gram-negative bacteria may mingle as well. The treatment should be started according to the result of the cultures from the biopsies [2].

The full treatment of chronic osteomyelitis is difficult to define, because relapses are frequent and after a very aggressive treatment, it may occur after months or years. After intensive attempts for a full treatment, sometimes the extremity-threatening surgical operation, occasionally a long-term treatment with toxic and expensive antibiotics is required.

Surgical intervention may be necessary to obtain culture material, and for the subtraction of sequestra, for removal of necrotic tissue and dead matter [10].

In 1995, Dr. Charles Lautenbach performed the **Lautenbach operation** for the first time. Dr. Lautenbach had been using this method in the treatment of chronic osteomyelitis for 30 years. From November 1995 until the end of 1998, the Sheffield Limb Reconstruction Service healed 17 patients by using the Lautenbach method. With all of the patients being male, the infection durations were 12.5 years. The method consists of the debridement of the dead bone, piercing the medullary canal, soft tissue debridement and the insertion of irrigation tubing. The main difference between the irrigation method and this method, is caused by the dispersion of the antibiotics in it. In traditional methods, the antibiotics are constantly dispersed; unfortunately, this means that the medullary canal is directly washed. Whereas in the Lautenbach method the antibiotics become injected once in every 4 hours, until a new instillation is needed, it remains in the cavity, it washes the tissues, are then are discharged.

Other advantages of the system:

- To provide the most appropriate concentration of the antibiotics in the area of the infection, 2 or more couples of lumen tube are used.
- For the control of the organisms, samples are taken from fluid of the washed medullary canals; and according to their susceptibility, the antibiotics are adjusted.
- Without a systematic side effect, a high dose of antibiotics can be dispensed through tubes. The antibiotics are dispensed only if the patient shows the systematic effects of the disease.
- For the evaluation of the course of the healing and the treatment, sinus dimensions can be taken.

The irrigation should be continued for at least 3 and at most 6 weeks. Before the tubes are removed, the criteria that are expected to be achieved are the following:

- Clean washing water
- Zero cavity dimensions
- In the washing water samples taken in sequence, no breeding of organisms should be observed
- Stable blood parameters [14].

3.2. Tuberculosis osteomyelitis

Primarily it is seen among adults, and the occurrence among children is rare. While in almost all of the cases *Myobacterium tuberculosis* is the agent, in rare cases atypical mycobacteria are reported to be the cause. There may be fever or not. However, patients with fever whose cause is unknown and with asymptomatic bone lesion should always be kept in mind. Although any bone can be involved, 50% of the cases are in the spine (50% thoracic, 25% cervical, 25% lumbar), 12% in the pelvis, 10% in the hip and femur, 10% in the knee and tibia, 7% in the ribs, and 2% in the ankle, shoulder, elbow or wrist, and in 3% more than one region is involved. In the diagnosis, chest radiography, tuberculin skin test and needle biopsy are used. As given in the treatment of lung disease, the regime is one composed of 9 to 12 months of isoniazid, rifampin, pyrazinamide, and ethambutol. Except for a very advanced disease, surgical treatment is rarely needed [10].

3.3. Newborn osteomyelitis

Newborn osteomyelitis is rare. Prematurity, low birth weight, another accompanying infection, blood transfusion, the presence of umbilical catheter may be considered as risk factors. Usually it is observed together in multiple bone and arthritis [3,10]. Because of nonspecific symptoms, the diagnosis may be delayed. As the most common S. aureus (> 90%), group B streptococci (especially in the postnatal 2-4 weeks) and enteric gram-negative bacilli may be the cause. There is no leukocytosis; ESR and CRP will have been increased. Mostly lytic bone lesions are seen in plain graphy. It may cause permanent disorders in joints and disturbance in the skeletal growth [3].

3.4. Osteomyelitis in sickle cell anemia

The susceptibility in the sickle cell hemoglobinopathies to bacterial infections has increased. During the sickling, due to microscopic infarcts, the blood invasion of intestinal microorganisms is facilitated. Besides, there is also splenic dysfunction. Of all the agents salmonella and gram-negative enteric bacilli factors (<70%), S. aureus are responsible. The diaphysis of the long bones, flat bones, the small bones of the hands and feet are often held. Acute vaso-occlusive crisis of the table is difficult to differentiate. It is difficult to distinguish the picture from an acute vaso-occlusive crisis. In both cases, there is fever, bone ache and leukocytosis. With MRI, one cannot distinguish an infection from an infarct. In a crisis attack, no response is obtained, needle aspiration and culture should be performed. A long-term (6-8 weeks) antibiotics treatment may be necessary for healing [3,9].

3.5. Traumatic osteomyelitis

Traumatic osteomyelitis develops as secondary in animal bites (especially due to Pasteurella multocida), and when blood is taken from newborns heel with needle sticking, during bone marrow aspiration, puncture injuries (especially when standing by *Pseudomonas* or by *Pseudomonas* through any injury somewhere) and due to open fractures including osteomyelitis. As *Aeromonas* is an unusual type of bacteria causing osteomyelitis with contaminated water [10].

3.6. Postoperative osteomyelitis

Postoperative osteomyelitis may develop in the process that follows the reduction of closed fractures, craniotomies, median sternotomies and other bone surgeries [10].

3.7. Multifocal osteomyelitis

Postoperative is mainly multifocal. Drug addiction may cause multifocal osteomyelitis. The scanning of multifocal hot spots on the bone may reveal multiple tumors, too [10].

3.8. Chronic recurrent multifocal osteomyelitis

This is observed in childhood and among young adults. Girls are more frequently affected. There are attacks that show similarity to osteomyelitis, recurrent high fever, swelling in bones, ache and radiologic visions. Palmoplantar pustulosis, psoriasis, arthritis, sacroiliitis, and inflammatory intestinal disease may occur together with the Sweet's syndrome. The SAPHO syndrome observed among adults (synovitis, acne, pustulosis, hyperostosis, and osteitis/osteomyelitis) is believed to be equivalent to the ones of childhood. Most frequently, the clavicle and the calcaneus are affected.

Bone cultures are sterile. Clear benefits of antibiotics cannot be shown, steroids and anti-inflammatory treatment is recommended. Although the etiology is unknown, the prognosis is positive [10].

3.9. Osteomyelitis in immunosuppressive hosts

Any organism (a rare one or superficial fungi) can cause osteomyelitis in these patients [10].

4. Possible nursing diagnoses

4.1. Collaborative problems in osteomyelitis

Infective emboli

Side effects of the antibiotics treatment (hematological, renal, hepatic) [15].

4.2. Nursing diagnoses

- Hyperthermia related to infections [16,17].
- Fluid Volume Deficiency Risk with regard to excessive fluid loss [16,17].
- Change in comfort depending on the infection, swelling, and hyperthermia process in the bone [15].

- Pain and discomfort, Physical Restriction of Movement associated with musculoskeletal disorders [16,17].
- Less Nutrition than the Body Requirements related to loss of appetite [15].
- Risk of Deterioration in Skin Integrity in relation to physical immobilization [15].
- Change in health condition, Anxiety in relation to hospitalization [16,17].
- Ache in relation to Inflammation/Infection [16,17].
- Risk of Injury in relation to immobilization because of spread of infections [16,17].
- Limited physical activity, Social Isolation in relation to therapeutic isolation [16, 17].
- Risk of Colonic Constipation due to immobility [15].
- Deficit in Entertainment Activities due to long-term hospitalization and insufficient mobility [15].
- Poor Nutrition: Change in Nutrition due to anorexia that is secondary to the infection process [15].
- Risk of Deficiency in Skin Integrity due to the mechanical irritation of the plaster/splint [15].
- Risk of Trauma depending on the Process of the Disease: Pathologic Fractures [15].

The situation is Risk of Ineffective Management of Therapeutical Regime due to the lack of knowledge on wound care, activity limitations, symptoms and findings of complications, follow-up of pharmacological treatment and care (check-up) [15].

5. Nursing management

The nursing of children who suffer from heavy musculoskeletal infections; for a wide range of evaluation it requires a multidisciplinary team approach that consists of as well as the hospital staff and services, pediatricians, orthopedists and infectious diseases specialists [18].

The main objectives of nursing care; to avoid possible complications, reduce pain, to inform the children and their families about the process of the disease and the treatment management. In the acute stage of the disease, restriction of movement may be observed in the affected joints. However, by supporting the affected joint, the child will be in a comfortable position. Cautiously and gently moving the patient will reduce the pain. Pain treatment will relieve the patient. Vital findings are taken and recorded. If important changes may occur in the measurements, then this is shared with the team members [19].

In the antibiotic treatment, careful observation should be performed; the vascular pathway area and the intravenous sets should be observed. Generally, several antibiotics are used together. One should consider that the used drugs are compatible with each other. The use of drugs that are not compatible should be avoided. For long-term antibiotics treatment, intermittent infusion devices or a central catheter (PICC) with peripheral input is used. The antibiotics therapy is often continued at home [19].

Isolation should be applied to children with an open wound. In wound care, the prescribed medicines are used. In addition, the insertion of antibiotic solutions into the wound care is very effective [19].

The received-removed fluid amount is continuously measured and recorded. Moreover, the wound drainage is also recorded. The state of healing of the wound tissue is evaluated and recorded [19].

To provide immobility, plaster is used and in such cases, routine plaster maintenance is performed [19].

The following are among nursing initiatives: Teaching the child to walk with crutches when necessary, ensuring that the child is kept away from slippery floors, preventing the child from moving in an uncontrolled manner during risk of insufficient mobility due to the plaster, and during the *Risk of Trauma* due to the dangers of walking with crutches [15,19]. Again, when necessary, supporting and observing the child during his/her walk and ensuring that the parents carry their children in or to safe environments. The family must be informed about the weight of the plaster and advised to adjust the body mechanics carefully while carrying the child or while giving position to him/her. The family must be warned not to take support from the plaster while lifting the child. Protecting the extremity in plaster from impacts is also among important nursing initiatives [19].

Risk of Deficiency in the Integrity of the Skin [15,19] as a result of the plaster applying a pressure on the skin surface and its being among important nursing initiatives, the nurses have to prevent the use of heating or cooling devices to dry the plaster because there is the risk of burning the skin under the plaster. Other nursing initiatives are as follows: observing the skin on the side of the plaster every day to see whether there is redness or not. Applying massage to these areas to prevent skin deficiencies. Placing cotton in these areas to prevent skin irritations. Explaining to the small children why they should not put pencils or other objects to the plaster. Elevating the extremity with plaster in order to prevent edema due to the pressure of the plaster. Following the extremity with plaster to see whether there are coldness, color change, edema, pain or numbness or not being able to check the pulse in the distal of the extremity and making neurovascular assessments [19].

Supporting the child to use his/her extremity without plaster in case of a *Lack of Self-Care* [15,19] as a result of the limitations in movement due to the plaster is also among nursing initiatives. It may be necessary to explain to the parents and to the child that the plaster will not prevent the daily care activities such as toilet need in the morning and general body cleaning [19].

Nursing Initiatives in *Lack of Entertainment Activities* [15,19] as a result of the limitations in movement due to the plaster are: Determining the entertainment activities of the child, ensuring that s/he plays chess or computer games, reads books, listens to music, draws pictures with the nurse or his/her parents or friends coming to visit if the child is bedbound [19].

In *Management of the Therapeutical Regime without Effects* [15,19], the important factors are, the maintenance of the plaster, the symptoms and findings of the complications, information on the use of helping-supporting devices. The relevant Nursing Initiatives are: If the plaster gets wet, its function will be disabled, therefore ensuring that the cleaning of the child with a piece of cloth is provided; keeping the plaster dry and clean; preventing the spill of food or drinks on the child by making him/her wear a pinafore; cleaning the pinafore if any food or drink is spilt. In case an area under the plaster itches, ensuring that cold air is blown is another nursing initiative. In case bad smell comes from below the plaster or the drainage area, its possibility of being a clue for an infection must be explained to the parents of the child. The knowledge that if the neurological and circulatory functions are broken, this might cause to permanent paralysis in extremities, to ischemia or damage in the nerves must be given to the parents. The information that, in case the plaster is near the perineum area, the plaster must not get dirty with the feces or the urine must be given to the parents as well. In addition, the parents must be informed about the situation when the plaster is removed, there might be dryness and peeling on the skin [19].

The affected area, whether in plaster or not is evaluated for color, edema, heat and sensitivity [19].

In the first stage of the treatment the child has no appetite. For a healthy diet, until the patient feels better, one is encouraged to consume high calorie liquids, fruit juice, ice cream and jelly. In order to have bone growth and healing, an adequate nutrition has to be provided [19].

After the treatment in the acute stage, the child will feel better. As a result of this, the appetite of the child will increase, and s/he will communicate socially. For this reason, the nurse may start entertaining and curative activities for the children in this period. However, these activities should be mostly in bed. Because resting of the child usually after the acute period is imperative. However, when isolation and bed-rest may not be required for a long term, moving in a wheelchair may be allowed [19].

The role of nurses is to provide information to patients and caregivers about the treatment, to support and to help for the treatment plan [14].

For providing the patient to go through the hospitalization period as comfortable as possible they are encouraged to share their fears and concerns [14].

Psychosocial evaluation leads to the possibility of self-recognition, coping mechanisms and to reveal the sources of motivation of the patient. This is for the creation of an appropriate and effective care-plan by the whole team. The patient should be informed about the contents of the processes, that the infection could not be eliminated successfully, risk factors like the development of a new infection, problems related to prolonged bed-rest and regarding a secondary reconstructive surgery. Patients that have become aware of being not sufficiently informed or being not included in the decision taking will be prone to depression. Regarding the information given, feedback from patients and caregivers should be taken. The preparation of the treatment facilities should be presented; and plenty of opportunities should be given to ask questions frequently [14].

Author details

Şenay Çetinkaya[1*] and Sibel Kuşdemir[2]

*Address all correspondence to: scetinkaya@cu.edu.tr

1 Adana School of Health, Çukurova University, Adana, Turkey

2 Nursing Department, Adana School of Health, Çukurova University, Adana, Turkey

References

[1] Çavuşoğlu H. Çocuk Sağlığı Hemşireliği Cilt 1. 5. Baskı. Ankara: Bizim Büro Basımevi, 2000; 351-362.

[2] Feigin R, Cherry J. Textbook of Pediatric Infectious Diseases. 4. Ed. NY: Saunders Company, 1998; 475-495.

[3] Hatipoğlu N, Yalçın I, Çocuk Enfeksiyon Hastalıkları. 1. Baskı İstanbul: Medya Tower Yayıncılık, 2007; 213-218.

[4] Gutierez K. Bone and Joint Infections in Children. North Am: Mosby, 2005; 780-794.

[5] Cantez T, Ömeroğlu R, Baysal S, Oğuz F. Çocuk Sağlığı ve Hastalıkları. İstanbul: Nobel Tıp Kitabevleri, 2003; 340-341.

[6] Dworkin P. Pediatrics. 2nd Ed. Malvern: Harwal Publishing Company, 1992; 243-244.

[7] Neyzi O, Ertuğrul T. Pediatri Cilt 2. 2. Baskı, İstanbul: Nobel Tıp Kitabevleri, 1993; 798-800.

[8] Öztuna V. Osteomiyelit patofizyolojisi ve tedavi prensipleri. Türk Ortopedi ve Travmatoloji Birliği Derneği Dergisi 2005; (4):63-71.

[9] Tabak F. İnfeksiyon Hastalıklarına Pratik Yaklaşımlar. 1. Baskı. İstanbul: İstanbul Medikal Yayıncılık, 2008; 123-141.

[10] Moffet H. L. Pediatric Infectious Diseases. 3rd Edition. Wisconsin: Lippincott Co. 1989; 422-432.

[11] Yalçın I, Salman N, Somer A. Pediatride Rutinler. 1st Edition. İstanbul: Medya Tower Tanıtım ve Yayıncılık Hizmetleri, 2007; 213-218.

[12] Yolbaş İ. Pediatrist Tanı Tedavi ve Reçete Kılavuzu El Kitabı. İstanbul: İstanbul Medikal Yayıncılık Ltd Şti, 2012; 123-125.

[13] Harik NS, Smeltzer MS. Management of acute hematogenous osteomyelitis in children. Expert Rev Anti Infect Ther. 2010 Feb; 8(2):175-181.

[14] Sims M, Trent JC, Lake S, Smith B, Hashmi MA, Saleh M.The Lautenbach method for chronic osteomyelitis: nursing roles, responsibilities and challenge Journal of Orthopaedic Nursing, 2001 November;5(4):198-205.

[15] Carpenito LJ. Handbook of Nursing Diagnosis. 7th Edition. Philadelphia, Newyork: Lippincott.Firdevs Erdemir (Çev. Edt). Hemşirelik Tanıları El Kitabı. İstanbul: Nobel Tıp Kitabevleri Ltd. Şti. ISBN: 975-420-020-3. 1999, pp. 491-492.

[16] Birol L. Hemşirelik süreci. 10. Baskı. İzmir: Etki Yayıncılık, 2011.

[17] Luxner K. Delmar's Pediatric Nursing Care Plans. 3rd Edition. NY: Thomson Delmar Learning 2005; 256-262.

[18] Copley LA, Kinsler MA, Gheen T, Shar A, Sun D, Browne R. The impact of evidence-based clinical practice guidelines applied by a multidisciplinary team for the care of children with osteomyelitis. J Bone Joint Surg Am. 2013 Apr 17; 95(8):686-693.

[19] Geçkil EA, Çetinkaya Ş, Cabar D. Çocuklarda Kas-İskelet Sistemi Hastalıkları, Yaralanmaları ve Hemşirelik Bakımı. In: Pediatri Hemşireliği. Conk Z, Başbakkal Z, Yılmaz HB, Bolışık B. (Edts). 17. Bölüm. Adana: Akademisyen Tıp Kitabevi. 2013. ss. 699-740.

Section 3

Pediatric Psychiatry

Chapter 5

The Psychological Problems Seen in the Children of Divorced Parents and the Nursing Approach Concerning These Problems

Şenay Çetinkaya and Emine Erçin

Additional information is available at the end of the chapter

http://dx.doi.org/10.5772/59166

1. Introduction

Millions of years have passed so far today since the appearance of mankind on earth, and people have been struggling quite a great deal in order to cope with life affairs for millions of years; yet, in today's context, it was in 2000 BC that they were able to comprehend the requirement of being spouses and parents. The proceeding/behaviour to be together or get together as husband and wife has been referred to as "matrimonial action/wedding", and this established relationship is called "marriage" [1].

Family is expressed as a social league with vital characteristics within a limited extent, which is based on an emotional commitment within a framework of solidarity that cannot be transferred to others [2].

A complete family is a community consisting of a mother, a father and children with mutual love, respect, support/solidarity and the sense of belonging to each other. Such a family is the fundamental factor in the emotional, social and moral development of the child. In sum, a complete family is a natural environment where the child is socialized in the broadest sense [3].

It is seen that the point of view/perspective on the concept of family began to change in the twentieth century. This different point of view on family also caused the parenthood to be considered as something independent of marriage. It has been stated that the differentiation of the point of view on marriage and having children when compared to the past is associated with the developments in technology [4].

A family established by "two different individuals" also has the potential of conflict and discrepancy along with it as the natural consequence of being two different individuals. It is too optimistic to expect the two different individuals with various personality traits who were raised in different environments to be always in harmony for years, since a family which is an institution considered to be a harbour against the challenges of life may, itself, sometimes turn into a a stormy ocean and create problems instead of solving them, in which case the spouses end up with the decision to terminate their association and get divorced, which is, today, experienced more and more in increasing numbers [1].

Besides the fact that the widowed woman or man, following her/his spouse's death, never confronts the various social and psychological negative consequences of having been divorced or widowed in this way within the society, she/he and her/his children even remember the deceased one with love and respect. The widowed spouse, when compared with a divorced one, can get married and start a family much more easily; thus, the child can regain a natural environment once again [3].

A child having an extramarital mother will never have had a complete family. Such being the case, the ability of the child to overcome the problems encountered as s/he grows up is dependent on the understanding/empathy the close environment around her/him will show towards her/his situation [3].

Different from the traditional families, parents in modern families focus all their financial and emotional sources along with all their attention and energy on raising children. For a woman, having a child becomes no more a conventionally inevitable role after marriage; instead, it becomes a period of personal decision/call and responsibility on the part of her. It is argued that the social changes, such as conceiving a child out of wedlock, or even the technological innovations like bearing a child through medium of sperm banks independent of the prospective father lead to a change in the point of view towards marriage and parenthood. It is now pointed out that a woman does not have a child just because she is married, and that having a child is not a marriage routine anymore but a decision independently made by the woman. Hence, it is also put forward that parenthood has lost its traditional relationship/ association with marriage. In the wake of such changes, it is also stated that the emotional value of the child, different from that of the traditional families, has increased even more. The most dramatic change of all the others within a family life throughout the twentieth century is said to have been the rapid increase in the divorce rate [4].

According to The National Survey of Family Growth (NSFG), the divorce rate in the USA is 3.6 per 1.000 population. The divorce rate is the highest in the males and females aged between 20-24, while this rate is the lowest in those aged between 35-39. Almost half of the marriages end up with divorce. The divorce rates have been on the increase since the beginning of 20th century, and particulary since 1970s. According to Brown et al.'s report (2008), the proportion of the nuclear families has declined from 85% to 69% for the last 30 years. Now 3 out of 10 children are living in single-parent homes [5].

It is seen that there has also been a great increase in the divorce rate in Turkey in recent years. According to the data of the State Statistics Institute (SSI), the divorce rate, starting from the years 1990s, have been on the increase to a great extent. The number of the married couples

http://dx.doi.org/10.5772/59166

getting divorced in 2011 increased at a rate of 1.3% in comparison to the previous year and reached 120.117.

The rough divorce rate was 1.62 per 1.000 population in 2011. Still, the divorce rates in our country are seen to be quite lower than those in several European countries. However, it is thought that the divorce rates seen to have increased particularly in big cities in recent years have been remarkable, and for this reason, it is important that divorce and the effects of divorce on individuals and the society be analyzed [4].

There are, undoubtfully, a number of reasons for the rapid increase in divorce rates. There are also various and major consequences of divorces, among which, as the sociologists and academicians put forth, is the case of shaking the society to its foundations. The very reason that it is the phenomenon/case shaking the foundations of the society is that it primarily affects the children, along with which the relationships between children and their parents, and between the parents are generally affected from this phenomenon in a negative way [3].

The case of a divorce is a blow inflicted on the self-confidence and self-respect of both the female and the male. However terrible the marriage is, the emptiness/separation experienced in the wake of a divorce is a major problem to be overcome [1].

Divorce is not a process experienced only between spouses. Most of the couples who are divorced have children, as well; therefore, a divorce is also quite an important process for the child. It is pointed out that a divorce potentially brings with it a series of changes that may seriously affect the child. Here, the reason for using the term "potentially" is that divorce is not regarded as a process that will inevitably harm children [4].

The first step in this challenging process is to explain to the child what divorce means. Some parents find it unnecessary to inform their children about their intention of getting divorced, and the fact that the age of the child is younger confirms/justifies this behaviour. Whereas, nobody-whether they love their parents or not-never understand the reason why, when they wake up one morning, one of their parents disappears as if s/he never existed. No child deserves to be left to confront such a devastating behaviour. Such thoughtless behaviours or actions may lead to the fact that they make up/imagine things which are unreal in order to compensate the situation or make some sense out of this as well as reinforcing their sense of being rejected [1].

How to tell the child about the decision to get divorced:

- The parents should explain to their child about their decision to get divorced in a secure and familiar environment the child is used to and should act together in this if possible.
- They should be totally honest in explaining the matter and use a comprehensible language by considering their age.
- The children should be listened to when they ask questions, the answers given should be limited to what is asked about and no long explanations should be included.
- While parents are having a conversation with their child(ren), they should avoid any mutual argument, nor should they blame each other in front of the child.

- The child should never be asked to take sides in this matter, in other words, s/he should never be put in the position of a referee.
- Even if one of the parents feel hatred or rage against the other party, no negative criticisms or remarks about him/her should be made behind his/her back.
- The remarks or expressions likely to hurt the child or make him/her feel guilty should carefully be avoided.
- The child should be given detailed information as to where s/he will live after divorce, with which parent s/he is going to stay with, how often s/he can see the other parent and what sort of changes will take place in her/his life after all.
- A child should never be regarded as a fellow sufferer or a shoulder to cry on. Otherwise, such a responsibility will be too heavy on him/her, which may have future consequences. Remember that your task of being a parent to them remains the same; what they need is your parenthood.
- The fact that the divorce takes place only between the father and the mother should particularly be emphasized. "We are getting separated but we are always your parents" [6].

Divorce is both a judicial and a psychological and social process. It is the life-style that may be traumatic for children and is unavoidable for some marriages [2].

When taken as a judicial concept, divorce, to put it simply, is the termination of a marriage contract [1].

In the light of the thought-provoking/challenging facts about the act of divorce and the increasing data suggesting that the children of divorced parents are at more risk than the others in terms of experiencing developmental and psychological problems, more and more couples are beginning to question whether it would be right to disperse/separate the family or not. Some of them, by putting aside their personal desires, consider continuing their marriage until their kids grow up and leave home. The research results have suggested that staying together merely for the sake of their children rarely works. Sometimes staying together for this reason becomes more harmful for the children of those keeping together than the children of those getting divorced due to discrepancy. The researches have revealed that the children who have witnessed various discrepancies/disagreements-from purposefully keeping still/silent or continuous noisy clamor to demonstrating physical violence-become more awkward and unbalanced than the children of those who got divorced. In short, sometimes the only way that seems to solve the problem could be to end the marriage [1].

2. The clinical characteristics of a divorce

1. *The Divorce Process:* It was found that the determining factor associated with divorce was the emotional and behavioural problems of spouses, and that the quality of marriage, the socio-economic conditions, postpartum depression and demographic changes were not

the determinants for that matter. It was seen that divorce takes place within an average of 3-year-process in between the decision to divorce and the divorce itself. It was determined that the children of the families living together after divorce had more adaptation problems compared to those whose families get married again [7].

In the process of a divorce, the situation reaches the stage of acceptance after having gone through the psychological reaction phases which are developed against a sense of loss witnessed in deadly-ill patients, such as denial, anger, bargaining, and depression, as defined by Elisabeth Kübler-Roos. The children also undergo similar stages as their parents do [7].

2. *The Denial Stage of Divorce:* At this stage, the children cannot accept the experiences associated with the divorce. They do not want to accept the separation of their parents. They cannot believe that their father and mother can care for them anymore; instead, they would rather believe that their parents will reunite. At this stage, it is important that parents deal with their discrepancies between each other in a proper way without ignoring the issues agreed upon and be clear about the child care period, as well. The reactions of denial and avoidance exhibited by the child can be overcome through an open communication. If the parents and their child(ren) ever get stuck in the denial period, the child(ren) will, then, not even agree to get any support to proceed with her/his life. The denial is followed by the accusation phase. In this phase, the child is outraged with his parents due to the fact that they do not get back together again, that they destroyed her/his whole life and hampered the realization of their dreams [7].

3. *Bargaining Stage:* This stage is the one at which the child makes an effort to fix the damage done by changing his/her own behaviours. S/he starts trying to accomplish her/his lessons without com plaining or quits fighting her/his sister/brother. Her/his belief that the parent who deserted her/him will come back one day. The belief that her/his parent left because of her/his misbehaviour may continue until advanced ages [7].

4. *Depression Stage:* The child is commonly seen to be tired, sad and depressed in living environments, at school and at home, where s/he may have difficulty in controlling her/his feelings/emotions. This stage usually lasts for a short time and does not necessitate a clinical intervention [7].

5. *Acceptance Stage:* The fact that divorce is a proper solution for parents is ensured by showing that the divorced parents now have individually happier lives compared to the previous one they had together. It may sometimes be possible to reach this stage during young adulthood. In the process of the ending relationship, often more intense and complicated emotions occur. Reconciliation in the wake of a divorce does not mean a reunion. It is the process in which the painful and challenging aspects of the relationship are integrated through experience and are no more obstacles against proceeding with life. The old and sorrowful processes are settled and the journey to the areas of new relationships goes on [7].

The researches carried out among children suggest that children do not accept the case of divorce; instead, they prefer a miserable marriage to a divorce [2].

The relationship of any child with her/his mother-father, in the first years of her/his life in particular, is of great importance. On the other hand, divorce is, doubtlessly, rather a challenging and stressful process for both children and their parents. Considering it from the child's side, the child will no more be able to reach the two people equally s/he has been mostly dependent on up to that time, that is, her/his parents, and her/his world will split up in a sense. Divorce, besides the changes taking place in the relationship of the patients, is quite important in terms of the parental roles of the divorced couples. When we analyze divorce in terms of parents, we encounter several problems to be coped with, such as re-building a new life following the divorce, developing new ways of contact with both the ex-spouse and the children, and additionally, the financial hardships occurring in the life of the divorced mother and the changes in social relationships [4].

One of the psychological variables that may cause a risk for the divorce of parents is the life satisfaction. Life satisfaction comprises the cognitive aspect of the concept of subjective well-being used as a synonym with happiness in the field of positive psychology. Accordingly, the subjective well-being (SWB) has two dimensions as the emotional/affective dimension consisting of positive and negative emotions and the cognitive dimension known as life satisfaction. Life satisfaction is also the cognitive judgement and evaluations made by the individual regarding her/his life. The conducted studies suggest that as the positive relationships of the adolescents with their parents increase along with the increase in the positive attitudes of a mother-father, commitment to parents and the socio-economic level, so does the life satisfaction escalate with such aspects. Thus, the familial variables are the important determinants of an adolescent/pubescent life satisfaction, and the changes within the family structure, like divorce, may affect the children's quality of life and the ways of perceiving their lives as is true for all the members of the family, as well [8].

It may be expected that the change in the life-style and circumstances also affect a child's life satisfaction in a negative way. As a matter of fact, the limited number of studies analyzing the life satisfaction of the children with divorced and undivorced parents show that the life satisfaction and general well-being levels of the children coming from broken families are lower than those coming from complete families. To sum up, the separation or the divorce of a child's parents causes a striking disadvantageousness due to the challenging life experiences brought to children's lives in terms of both their psychological developments and life satisfaction [8].

Another point to be highlighted is the extreme tolerance the mother shows towards her child in order to compensate the separation with her/his father, which may pave the way for the development of different behavioural problems in the child. For this reason, the balance should be maintained well, and the children should not be allowed to experience such borderline problems. In the wake of separation or divorce, the parents should not speak out against each other, nor should they reflect any problem they may be having with each other on the child. Such is the case commonly seen in divorced families, which may bring major problems with it. The child should also be allowed to see her/his parent living away from her/him frequently (unless there is some problem) and thus, the communication between the child and the other parent should be sustained [1].

http://dx.doi.org/10.5772/59166

Following the divorce, the relationship of the child with both of her/his parents will differ as compared to that in the past. After the divorce, the child will start living with this single parent, which is usually the mother in such cases. Therefore, major changes take place in the relationship between the child and the father who has left home after divorce. These major changes occurring in the child's and the parents' lives in the wake of the divorce are seen in a number of areas, such as the frequency of the meetings with both the parent living together with the child and the other parent living away, and the parents' responsibilities towards their child(ren) as well as fulfilling the tasks regarding them. Thus, it is required that both the mother and the father, after having been divorced, adapt to the new circumstances while maintaining their relationship with their children and re-structure this relationship for their new life-style [4].

Many children but the little ones know what divorce means due to the fact that the termination of marriages today is a commonly-seen incident. If there is tension and unhappiness within a family, it is greatly likely that the children within that family circle become aware of the fact that something is going wrong. Within the families where fightings, particularly the physical violence and alcoholism are often seen, the children learn to read the psychological states of their parents without any awareness. They can find the best time to approach an angry or an unhappy parent by starting from various details. In the same way, they know when to get away from the clamour. Even knowing something more or less about divorce and witnessing the continuous fight between their mother and father do not prepare most of the children to the news that her/his parents are separating ways or getting divorced. Once the incident breaks out-which often happens with one of the parents leaving home-the child literally gets shocked. If the child has been kept away from her/his parents fights up to that time, s/he even experiences a greater shock. Drifting away from a parent, even if it may be an abusive one, horrifies a child. It is natural for a child to miss the parent who left the family. The separation of the parent does not annihilate the children's sense of commitment [1].

The best time to explain the case of divorce to children should be at least one week before the day when one of the spouses will leave home, since the children will have quite a lot of questions and worries preoccupying their mind once they have got the news [1].

Divorce may occur as a major transformation in a child's life. If, for instance, the child has a chronic disease, the divorce in question poses an extra load/burden on the stress experienced in struggling with the disease. Witnessing the loss of love between parents, the abandonment of matrimonial obligations by parents, getting used to travelling between two different homes and the feeling of daily absence of a parent while living with the other one all cause new familial circumstances for the child. Divorce is a turning point in a child's life, since the ongoing life has changed to a considerable extent [5].

Brown et al. (2008) assume that 20-30% of the children and adolescents in the USA suffer from chronic diseases. The parents of the children with severe or chronic diseases may confront a higher risk of divorce. The data regarding the effect of the diagnosis of a child with a chronic disease on the marriage relationship are inadequate. As the result of the research, the reasons supporting a negative impact involve the communication problems, increased role tension, decreased relationship satisfaction and spending less time with a parent [5].

Syse et al. (2010) did not find any difference in the divorce rates between the couples who had a child with cancer and those who had a child with no cancer. They found out that when the educational levels of the mothers having children with cancer were higher than the average, the divorce rates in those parents proved to be higher, as well [5].

The age of the child, the gender, parental attitudes, educational status of parents, the socio-economic level of the family, the parents' professions, the number of sisters-brothers and the success status of the child are the factors affecting anxiety. The situations causing anxiety/worry in little children pave the way for the psychological reactions in the advanced ages. The ongoing disputes/conflicts between the separated parents even after the divorce may give rise to the occurrence of anxiety in the child. Anxiety may manifest itself in children in the form of different reactions. Some children withdraw in order to avoid any worrying situation and abstain from joining any groups of their peers, while others develop defense mechanisms, such as retreat, rejection, repression and projection [2].

3. The adaptation of children after divorce can be analyzed in 2 stages

1. *The short-term adaptation of the child towards divorce:* This is the adaptation process within the first few years. The existence of negative factors, such as the conflicts experienced by the child within the family, the lack of communication between parents, economic difficulties and stress factors, makes it hard for the child to adapt to the new stage in her/his life. Having been influenced very negatively in cognitive, emotional, social and behavioural ways during this period, the children enter a short period of mourning/lamentation against this process of change within the family. In consequence of the inner conflicts they experience, they may suffer from fear, sorrow, anger, guilt, loneliness, rejection, sense of being unloved, and physical problems like stomachache, headache and chest pain, and psychosomatic disorders like oversleeping and overeating, particularly within the first year following the divorce [9].
2. *The long-term adaptation of the child towards divorce:* This period starts after the first two years following the divorce and may continue until adulthood. In general, the adaptation to the process of change experienced within the family is provided in this process. If, in this process, the conflicts between the mother and father continue, the children's adaptation to this period becomes challenging, as the result of which there may be emotional and behavioural problems exhibited by the child [9].

The vulnerability that a divorce creates on the child is associated with, particularly, age, gender, the stress level experienced within the family in the divorce process and whether the parental functions are sufficiently fulfilled or not [9].

It was reported that the most important factor regarding the child's adaptation to this new state was his/her age at the time of divorce. Children, either at very young ages or in late adolescence, are influenced less by the long-term negative effects of divorce when compared with the other periods of age [9].

http://dx.doi.org/10.5772/59166

The children of the divorced parents experience a much more challenging process during adolescence when several developmental changes are being experienced, such as acquiring a social, sexual and occupational identity, having the capacity of getting independent, acquiring competence and being able to establish close relationships. It is reported that in comparison to the adolescents in the undivorced families, the risk of getting expelled from school, antenuptial conception and exhibiting antisocial actions increased 2-3 times more in those with the divorced parents [10].

The comparative studies conducted on the matter suggest that the children with divorced or separated parents, compared to those living with their families, develop a distrustful way of commitment towards their parents, and that their tendency to exhibit instant rage, constant rage, self-accusation, desperateness, depression and the tendency to commit suicide is higher than the others. The social adaptation, self-esteem and psychological resilience levels of those with divorced parents were found to be lower [8].

While some research results suggest that boys are much more influenced by a divorce when compared to girls, other research results show that this is just the other way round. In the study conducted by Aslıhan (1998) with a group of children belonging to broken and complete families, it was determined that male students had a higher level of anxiety in comparison to female ones. A significant difference was determined between the levels of anxiety in terms of the genders of children whose parents were not divorced. No significant difference was ascertained between the self-esteem levels in terms of the anxiety level ages of the children with divorced/separated parents [2].

As is seen, it is impossible to make generalizations as to how the act of divorce influences children, since each divorce case is indeed a unique, complex and multi-faceted event. However, despite all, the psychologists and academicians claim that several generalizations can be made as to how a divorce may affect a child by considering her/his age at the time of divorce [3].

4. Reactions to divorce that are unique to age

4.1. Between birth-age one (age of confidence/trust)

- They constantly show bad tempers.
- It is difficult for them to adapt to a change.
- Babies and those in their infancy feel the pain whenever they are separated from their parents.
- They do not feel themselves secure/safe during the times when the parents are together or when they feel the changes in the emotional state of one of the parents. They may react to such changes by crying, clinging or showing bad tempers [11].

4.1.1. What do they need?

- The environmental changes should be limited as much as possible.
- Parents must be particular about setting arranged time for their children's nutrition and sleep.
- A great deal of closeness should be shown as much as possible, both verbally and physically.
- Parents should spend a good deal of time by cradling, holding, caressing their babies and singing songs to them.
- Babies should be often allowed to contact with both parents.
- A parent should be able to communicate with the other parent about what to do in order to act in accordance/consistently.
- Once the baby utters her/his first word or takes her/his first step, the parent involved should share this experience with the other one.
- The new-born babies, particularly the premature ones, are oversensitive. It is highly necessary not to shout or fight when the baby is close.
- A calm/soothing tone of voice should be used while speaking to the other parent at the time of changing hands in holding the baby [11].

Thus, for instance, it is argued that a nurseling does not suffer much from a divorce. The reason for this is considered as the inability of the nurseling to understand the dispute between parents, and besides being incapable of taking sides, s/he is usually left to her/his mother's care [3].

The thought that the babies in their infancy will be least influenced by a divorce with the assumption that s/he is yet unaware of many things is wrong. In the babies at these ages were prominent changes in behaviours observed after divorce. The most striking ones were crying and crying jags, sleep disorders and malnutrition, and the loss of interest in toys. Hence, even at this age group, the couples getting separated after a divorce should do a good planning to share their responsibilities for the baby and come together with him/her. In the meantime, they should never attempt to fight or argue in front of the baby [12].

4.2. Between the ages of one-three (the world revolves around them)

- Change is hard/challenging for them.
- They are scared of separation and the visits from one parent's home to another's could be rather traumatic.
- They may show bad tempers or may cry for the other parent.
- They may want you stay with them and never get out of their sight, and when you attempt to go, they may desperately cling to you.
- They may suffer from such problems as falling asleep or staying awake the whole night [11].

4.2.1. *What do they need?*

- As the kids at this age range have no accurate comprehension of time, the separations may appear to be dreadful to them and seeing her/his parent that separated a week later may feel like eternity to him/her. That's why, a kid at this age gets into a tantrum and cries while getting apart from the other parent.
- Being in contact with both of the parents may help the kid's fears of separation diminish.
- Make sure that s/he fully trusts your love and that you will meet his/her needs.
- Show him/her that you understand her/his yearning/longing for the other parent. Show him/her when to meet or call the other parent again by using the calendar.
- Hug him/her with love to make the separation easier and tell her/him that you will always be there and love him/her.
- Set predictable, reliable boundaries and prescribe coordinated programs.
- Ensure that s/he goes to bed at the exact hour in both homes.
- Reading him/her the same bed-time story and letting him/her sleep with the most beloved blanket and toy of his/hers could be useful [11].

4.3. Between the ages of three-five (age of curiosity)

- Fear of being abandoned.
- Feeling guilty, angry, nervous, scared, sad and confused.
- Being anxious/concerned about whether or not they are safe or loved.
- Blaming themselves for the divorce.
- Believing that their hostile thoughts or bad tempers caused their parents to split up.
- Dreaming about the reunion of their parents.
- Making futile efforts in order to unite their parents.
- Extreme obedience.
- Thinking like "I'm not good enough" or "I'm an evil person".
- Having difficulty in making visits between homes.
- Returning to behaviours, such as wetting the bed, thumbsucking, etc.
- Anxi4ety may lead them towards masturbation, whereas some others may develop tantrums or experience sleep disorders.
- Since the concept of continuity in little kids has not yet been developed, they may repeatedly ask when their mother or father will come back home although you have told them you will not be living together anymore [11].

The preschoolers may be seen as those who are most intensely influenced by a divorce. The kids of these ages consider themselves as the focus of attention in life and thus, within their family circle. This notion prompts them to the feeling of guilt, with the presumption that *they* are responsible for a possible divorce. With the child's mind, they may tussle with the ideas like "mum and dad are fighting because I do not behave well, and they got separated because of me…". Ultimately, the most commonly seen problems emerge once again, such as wetting the bed, thumbsucking, finding the shelved and already-worn out teddy bear to sleep together with. Such behaviours reveal the extent to which the child is tormented with the insecure, defenseless feelings of neediness [12].

4.3.1. What do they need?

- Talk to your child about your divorce issue and let them ask questions about it.
- If the kid repeatedly asks whether or not her/his mother/father is coming back, just answer him/her calmly and tell him/her that you have already got divorced and her/his mother/father is now living in a new place.
- Tell him/her when s/he could see the other parent.
- Kids express their emotions indirectly. They need help in order to express their emotions properly. (Parents may help their kids by reading them decent stories about other kids whose parents got divorced.)
- When you see your child sad or worried, ask her/him to draw or paint pictures regarding their emotions and thoughts on what has been happening. Hand them baby dolls and puppets to help them cope with their emotions. (Watch them while they are playing games and listen to their speech. In this way, you can get clues as to how they adapt to the case of divorce).
- Teach your children new words about emotions. (Use your daily experiences as the chance to define the emotions).
- The little kids need explanations as to the fact that it is not they who have caused a crisis within the family and that it is not their task to solve it.
- Show them you love them with a physical closeness and ensure them that you will undertake any care they need any time.
- If they are still dreaming about the reunion of the family, tell them that their wish is natural and ok but impossible to come true again.
- In order to prepare your child for the change between homes, play games with them related to these visits to both homes. (By placing chairs in two separate rooms, tell your child that one of the rooms belongs to her/his mother and the other to her/his father. While you are performing imaginary visits with your child between the rooms, tell her/him what to do and what to bring with her/him during these visits. Make it a fun game to play in order to make the real visits become sort of fun for the child) [11].

In this age and during the time until preschool period, if the child has been left under the negative impact of the main divorce in particular, the negative behaviours to be observed in the child are fear, stubbornness, sleep disorders, poor feeding, bed wetting, stuttering, etc. [3].

4.4. Between the ages of six-eight (age of sparse teeth)

- Kids feel themselves split in two.
- They may blame themselves for the divorce.
- They assume they will be deprived of food and toys or will be neglected by their parents.
- They usually feel abandoned/deserted.
- They may have feelings of rejection, loss, and the contradiction as to whom they should be loyal to, along with the feelings of guilt.
- They have the anxiety that they have lost the separated parent eternally, and they get scared of the idea of another person taking their place.
- They often cry and show bad tempers.
- They feel emptiness and have difficulty in concentrating at school.
- They may regard the divorce as a battle requiring them to take sides.
- They long for the parent living away from home and try to unite them again, and they even write notes full of love, pretending to be the other parent sending the note to his/her spouse.
- They do not state that they are stressful /tense. The problems caused by divorce result from several nervous attitudes, such as nose-picking, hair-twisting, making face/frowning, stuttering, nail-biting and chewing pencils, etc. They may withdraw cry, get furious and aggressive or become extremely placid/ meek.
- If the cause of divorce is not explained to them, they will find a way in their own way to get it explained. Since they are still unable to comprehend that there are two sides to both of the stories, they may totally put the blame on a single parent. If, for instance, one of the parents start seeing somebody else right after the divorce, then s/he may be the one to be blamed for [11].

No matter how understanding they may seem towards the reasons for the divorce explained to them, the kids at this age, in fact, subside into the intense feeling of loss for the matter involved. Nevertheless, the kids at this age, contrary to the little ones, do not take the blame on themselves but put it on their parents. They feel rage against their elders, get disappointed and consider themselves rejected. From time to time, with the notion that they have to take sides, either that of the father or the mother, they may exhibit behaviours like bearing a grudge against the other parent. Almost all of them have trouble at school after the divorce, and their success at school declines, as well [12].

4.4.1. What do they need?

- Since their skills to think logically has not yet been improved, it may be useless to try to make cool and reasonable explanations to them.
- They need help in defining their emotions and expressing them verbally. (Look through the magazines with your child. Mark the sad, angry, scared or happy faces and comment on what that person might be feeling at that time).
- The children at this age would like to make their parents pleased. (Since they may be wishing to be loyal to both sides, it is of utmost importance not to talk negatively against the other parent).
- Early school age kids need the assurance/guarantee that they be taken care of and their needs be met. (Make them sure that they are safe and that you have plans to protect her/him against any vice.).
- If you need to cut down on expenses due to financial problems, explain to your kid that they will always have a secure place to eat and live in.
- The kids at this age are in need of physical closeness/affinity. (Hug/hold them when their peers are not around) [11].

It is best to explain to the kids at this age the reasons for the divorce without any lies in it. They should be treated like an adult rather than like a child. Separately, since many children tend to hide this family issue from their friends and teachers, their teachers must definitely be informed about the issue, at least, in order to avoid the problems that may occur at school [12].

4.5. Between the ages of nine-twelve (age of success)

- The processes of divorce and remarriage is particularly difficult for the children at these ages.
- They begin to understand the family/parental relationships and are more sensitive to conflicts.
- Divorce causes anger and shame in many children, and the changes to take place makes them really anxious. (Anxiety is reflected through their behaviours, such as bad tempers or challenges they encounter in their lessons).
- They may fight with their peers or just keep away from them.
- They may start having nightmares.
- They may get offended or nervous without knowing the underlying cause. (They may feel a sense of anger, pain, anxiety and weakness).
- Emotions like the feeling of loneliness, loss and deprivation may lead to depression or other emotional problems.

- Since the children at this age distinguish everything as black or white, they are quite sensitive to the pressures put by their parents with respect to taking sides in the matter.
- They become worried/anxious about their parents. (They may try to substitute the parent who left and behave as if they were mature enough to handle things).
- They understand the psychological states /moods of their parents more easily and wonder whether they will be able to take care of their children or not [11].

For all that, a child is influenced by the divorce during the school age at most. S/he has begun to understand the discrepancy between her/his mother and father and to take sides between them already. The divorce results in losing her/his trust/confidence in her/his father or mother, or both [3].

4.6. Between the ages of thirteen-eighteen (the age of enraged hormones)

- During this period, it may be rather painful and shocking for a child to see their parents divorce.
- They may show reluctance in getting involved in emotional relationships. Besides, with the feeling of having been deserted, they may get away from home often and spend more time with their peers.
- They experience sense of loss and anger/rage.
- They may be scared of getting hurt, or assume that their own marriage, one day, will also fail and they may be afraid of repeating the same mistakes their parents made.
- The financial matters and the psychological states of their parents worry them a great deal.
- They may have difficulty concentrating on their lessons at school.
- They may complain about physical health problems or experience chronic fatigue.
- They may easily sink into a depression because of the fact that family is now no more a safe harbour to rely on.
- Inappropriate/unbalanced behaviours can be observed in the children who have difficulty in understanding the divorce or accepting this fact. (Fleeing from school, making friends with children exhibiting improper actions, using alcohol, committing suicide, etc...) [11].

The adolescents who are affected by the divorce at most are those who cannot find a peaceful home in their new lives. If there was an uncomfortable environment prior to the divorce which may have psychologically shocked the adolescent, then the impact of divorce may increase more and more. The adolescent may consider himself/herself as the cause of divorce. S/he creates the psychological problem with which s/he assumes that his/her parents quarreled because of his/her actions and, therefore, it is s/he who has caused this separation [13].

4.6.1. What do they need?

- The children in this period require proper ways to reveal their emotions and also need encouragement from their parents.
- It is important to arrange family gatherings and have one-to-one conversations with both of the parents.
- Writing poetry, painting, keeping a diary, writing and sending letters to the parents may help them express their urge to throw things away or hide them.
- You should be honest to your child about your divorce without giving too much detail. Never ask them to take sides.
- You must never rely on them for a psychological support.
- Encourage them to spend time with their peers. You can also support their friends's visits to both homes.
- While the calendar is being marked for mutual visits or some sorts of changes are being made, the opinions of the children of this period should also be taken into account, however, the final decision should be made by the parents.
- It is indeed a difficult situation for the children aged 11 and above to observe their parents get interested in the opposite sex and to see them get engaged in an emotional relationship, because they have already started to be aware of their own sexuality. Thus, before showing any physical affinity/ intimacy towards the person you are interested in right in front of your child, spare some time for them to get to know that person and get used to him/her.
- You should continue setting clear, reasonable and steady boundaries without letting him/her take shelter in the other parent's home by running away from house chores and responsibilities [11].

This is the age group in which divorce is mistakenly thought to have the least impact on children. Whereas, at this age, the child who already carries the burden of puberty/ adolescence with him/her becomes faced with an additional stress factor with the divorce of his/her parents. Their initial reactions are generally centered on starting to behave more distant towards their parents, spending most of their time with their friends rather than their parents and feeling, in their environment, ashamed of this incident experienced within the family [12].

Female children usually give more sensitive reactions compared to male ones. The increasing interest towards the opposite sex due to the loss of confidence experienced against their parents and having a sexual experience at an early age as the result of confiding in a protective male companion are the possible consequences to occur in this respect. Male children, on the other hand, show more aggressive reactions [12]. The negative behaviours exhibited by the children at this age are failure at school, telling lies, stealing, sexual perversion, etc.. Moreover, starting from this period, the child begins to encounter various problems that cannot be resolved only by his/her parent and him/herself, against which s/he may be carried away with the sense of insufficiency [3]. The most important outcome to be expected and be careful about is their ending up in a youth detention center due to their tendency to commit crimes at an early age. Further problems in both of the genders, such as becoming drug addicts and giving harm to themselves should also be taken into account [12].

As is seen, it is almost impossible to find out in families with children the ideal age of the child during the period of divorce. The separation of parents will bring with it the problems considered to be rather intense for any child at any age group, since the dream about a "holy and healthy family" remains the same for any child, from infancy to adolescence [12].

4.7. The grown-up children (what would i like to do?)

- Those who left home, and those who even have kids have difficulty in understanding the divorce of their own parents. They keep asking, "why now?".
- Since divorce has undermined their feeling of confidence, they may avoid making long-term promises.
- Considering that life has no guarantee, and since they are scared of being betrayed or deserted, they turn to interdependent relationships and choose the people who will need them most so that they can never be abandoned.
- Those living away from home may feel anxious and angry as to which parent they are going to spend their vacation with.
- The married ones may question the stability of their own marriage due to their parents' current situation.

4.7.1. What do they need?

- You should tell them that both parents contribute to the problems within the marriage, that it is hard after all to continue like that and people can change in time.
- Still, it will be your responsibility to give them some hope to be able to establish positive relationships and to sustain their own marriage and explain to them how important it is to have communication and agreement and to solve problems in marriage.
- It is necessary that you not complain about the other parent and not force the grown-up child to take sides in this matter by blaming the other one.
- If the other parent is not communicating with your child and not visiting him/her regularly, do not force him/her to establish a relationship with the child, because it is important that s/he develop their relationships without your influence.
- You should tell your child that you will maintain your relationships with her/him and your grandsons/granddaughters, and that you will continue their school activities and other activities, as well. You should also talk to them about how you will spend the vacations together [11].

The Reactions to the Loss of the Beloved Parent						
	Dysphoric Reactions		**Reactions to the other Parent**		**The Expressive Reactions**	
	Pain and hopelessness	Comforting one's self	Dependency	Fear of Loss	Anger/Rage	Restlessness
Infancy	Sorrowful, crying, mourning, apathy	Thumbsucking, Caressing and holding the toys	Clinging	Concern /worry about separation	Similar anger	Agitation
Preschool period	Crying (yet, decreased), sadness, withdrawal	Masturbation	Clinging, desire to be taken care of.	Concern /worry about separation	Revealing/ expressing anger and rage in games	Agitation
Middle Childhood	Crying, sadness		Clinging, whining, childish speech, independence	School fobia	Disobedience, fleeing from school, committing crimes	Restlessness, decline in school success
Puberty/ Adolescence	Tearful state, sadness, fatigue			School fobia	Rebellion, sexual acts, belligerence, rudeness, drug abuse, use of alcohol, escape from home	Restlessness, decline in school success

Table 1. The Reactions Shown by Children Against the Loss of the Beloved Parent After Divorce

Parents should try to learn how to approach their children. Even though they decide to get a support from a mental health specialist, the child who particularly fails to accept the separation of his/her mother and father or rejects it may, of course, refuse to get such a support. In order to enable their child to adapt him/herself to the divorce process, parents should be able to do the following:

- To make their child understand what it means for a family to live under the conditions unique to themselves and what divorce means in that sense, which should be done together and without ever blaming each other.
- To tell them that it is not their fault when parents get divorced in accordance with their age, and to explain with tangible/concrete expressions in what way it will affect them.
- To encourage the children in maintaining a happy and warm relationship with the other parent and to do his/her best in this respect.

- To make their children believe that they will always be loved and taken care of in the best way and to do the best in this respect.
- To maintain the relationship with the ex-spouse as smoothly as possible. To co-operate with each other in the issues involving the child. If this is not possible, it is better not to reflect any problems to the child.
- To encourage the children in asking for assistance and guidance from other people in their lives or from the specialists [7].
- Motivate your children in expressing their emotions. Avoid your impulse to tell him/her how to feel. Your child may withdraw and once s/he does that, the possibility of sharing the emotions diminishes.
- Avoid attempting to get engaged in any legal battles as to how your child shall stay with which parent. Such court issues may cause the child to consider the future from an insecure perspective. Do not separate the sisters/brothers from each other unless one of the children in his/her puberty period clearly states that he wants to live away from her/his sister/brother [14].

5. The nursing approach to the children of divorced families

Children may require a professional health team in order to minimize their negative emotions and misunderstandings and to get help in trying to cope with the problems experienced in the wake of the divorce. The psychiatric nurses within this team have a major position due to the fact that they can directly reach children and know the dynamics within the family and are aware of the way the child is influenced [15].

The main purpose of the nurses working in this field is to determine the high-risk groups within the society and improve their ability to cope with problems and aid them to manage the state of crisis they encounter. In this context, they deal with the problems experienced by the children of the divorced parents by using the nursing process [15].

The first stage of this approach is the one known for the term "determining the situation"-the stage where the data that could form the basis to the care of the individual are collected. The second stage comprises the analysis of the collected data and the determination of the nursing diagnosis through the interpretation of the data, while the third stage consists of the plan of attempts/interventions prepared for the problems of the patient and based on the knowledge and ability of the nurse to make a decision. The fourth stage, on the other hand, is the stage at which this plan is put into effect. The final stage is the one at which there are reviews as to whether the attempts have resolved the individual's problems or not and an evaluation is performed with respect to it [15].

The problems experienced by the children of the divorced families were formulated by using the nursing diagnoses determined by NANDA (North America Nursing Diagnosis Association), and the nursing attempts in accordance with these diagnoses have been explained [15].

The problems experienced by the children of the divorced parents can be dealt with the following nursing diagnoses:

1. Situational Low Self-Esteem
2. Change in interparental processes
3. Insufficiency in individual coping
4. Failure in Communication [15].

6. Situational low self-esteem

Self-esteem is one of the four elements of the self-concept and is the sum of an individual's skills, the value attributed to himself/herself and to others by him/her, the skill to be able to overcome hardships, and the feelings and thoughts s/he has in regard to respect for others. The development of a healthy self-esteem in children is dependent on their closeness/ affinity to the most significant figures in their lives, who are their parents. The children of divorced families have witnessed the separation of the two most important people in their lives and have been emotionally affected by it through experiencing the feeling to lose them. For this reason, such can be the case in a child who once had a positive self-esteem but experienced negative emotions as the result of their parents' divorce [16]. The objectives and the general nursing attempts to be performed for the diagnosis dealt with as the situational low self-esteem are as follows:

Objectives

1. The ability of the child to express the emotions s/he has felt regarding the divorce.
2. The ability of the child to sort/sequence the changes that the divorce brought into his/her life.
3. The ability of the child to express his positive and negative thoughts and the social areas s/he succeeds in [16].

Nursing Attempts

- The child is allowed to express his/her emotions about divorce through medium of emotion cards, pictures or puppet games.
- The changes that the divorce may bring into the child's life are explained through illustrative materials and the changes in the life of the child are discussed.
- The child is allowed to define himself/herself through various games s/he could be fond of according to the age group and to become aware of her/his positive traits via such activities; therefore, the advantages of sparing time for the activities s/he is talented in or does with delight, such as sports, music, etc., are discussed [16].

7. Change in interparental processes

Divorce causes a number of changes within the present family structure and functioning and also brings about the separation of the family members, leading to the formation of a single-parent family. The changes taking place in the life of the child along with his/her parents' divorce (Moving to another house, a new school, living in two different homes, spending less time with the parent, etc.) are the situations that are difficult to accept. All these transformations also cause a change in the interparental processes [17]. The objectives and the general nursing attempts to be performed for this diagnosis are as follows:

Objectives

1. The ability of the child to express and become aware of the changes/transformations s/he has experienced in the wake of divorce.
2. The ability of the child to reveal his/her emotions regarding the changes experienced.
3. The ability of the child to comprehend that there are different types of families.
4. The ability of the child to describe her/his emotions about the family members s/he is living with and those s/he is away from.
5. The ability of the child to arrange the frequency of the meetings with her/his parent living away [17].

Nursing Attempts

- The experiences of the child are discussed by making use of the books which describe the changes that the kids of the divorced families undergo. As the result of these changes, the emotions experienced by the child are discussed through the group process.
- By using the pictures illustrating different family types, the structure of a single-parent family is focused on, and the child is aided to reveal his/her feelings about this.
- By co-operating with the parents after divorce, the responsibilities undertaken by both parents in regard to the child's routine activities (Going to school, seeing the parent who lives apart from him/her,etc.) are reviewed, and the child is assisted to balance the frequency and period of the meeting with the separated parent.
- The child is encouraged to talk about his/her feelings and thoughts related to the parent living away from him/her [17].

8. Insufficiency in individual coping

With the divorce, the children experience the feeling of losing both their mother and father.

The fact that one of the parents leave home during this period and the changes in the new school environment, new friends and the house order make it difficult for the child to adapt himself/herself to these changes and they negatively affect their skill to cope with such issues [16]. In such a period of time, the objectives and the general nursing attempts to be performed for supporting the child in coping with the problems can be as follows:

Objectives

1. Allowing the child to become aware of the methods s/he uses in coping with the divorce and to express them.
2. Allowing the child to define the concept of problem solving and to sequence/sort the problem solving steps.
3. The ability of the child to comprehend the realtionships between problems, resolutions and emotions.
4. Allowing the child to become aware of the problems s/he can solve in his/her life and those s/he cannot.
5. Allowing the child to comprehend the ways of coping with problems that s/he is unable to solve [16].

Nursing Attempts

- The problems experienced by the child with respect to the divorce are reviewed, and the ways to cope with them while solving them are discussed.
- The best and the most proper method to cope with issues are stated to be problem solving ones, and by using the illustrated materials, the problem solving steps and their relationship with the emotions are discussed.
- How various issues encountered in his/her daily life can be resolved through the problem solving steps is discussed.
- Several cards on which the problems to be experienced by the children of the divorced parents are written are prepared, and the child is made to exercise the problem solving skills through games [16].
- The child is helped to understand that there may be problems in his/her life that s/he can solve as well as those s/he will be unable to solve. (Re-union/re-marriage of the parents, providing reconciliation between them, etc.).
- It is explained through the examples of real life events that people may get offended or enraged against the problems they are unable to solve; however, anger or rage can, of course, be expressed in a constructive way, as well [16].

9. Failure in social relationships

Divorce and the changes it brings along affect the social relationships in a negative way as well as the the child's interaction within the family circle [16]. The objectives and the general nursing attempts to be performed for this diagnosis are as follows:

Objectives

1. The ability of the child to share his/her feelings about the divorce with his parents.

2. Allowing the child to comprehend the importance of the regularity and permanency of the days when s/he is together with her/his parent living apart and the one living with her/him.

3. Allowing the child to take part in the events that may improve his/her social relationships [16].

Nursing Attempts

- Following the divorce, the importance of sharing feelings with parents is discussed, and the child is encouraged about the importance of sharing his/her emotions with his/her parents in that matter.
- Discussing with the child about the necessity and importance of establishing positive relationships with the parent living apart and the one living with him/her together. In this case, both parents are worked with in coordination, and the necessity of the quality time they spend together with their children and its positive effects on children are explained.
- The child is encouraged/motivated to participate in the activities s/he is interested in, both within and outside the school [16].

As a result, the nurses help the children of the divorced families cope with the crisis they experience in their lifetime by dealing with the problems the children undergo through the nursing process; thus, they can also assist the future generations to grow up as healthier and more conformable individuals that have acquired skills in coping with the problems of life [15].

Author details

Şenay Çetinkaya[1*] and Emine Erçin[2]

*Address all correspondence to: scetinkaya@cu.edu.tr

1 Adana School of Health, Çukurova University, Adana, Turkey

2 Nurse at Department of Psychiatry, Balcalı Hospital, Çukurova University, Adana, Turkey

References

[1] Türkaslan N. Boşanmanın Çocuklar Üzerine Olumsuz Etkileri ve Bunlarla Başetme Yolları (The Negative Impacts of Divorce on Children and the Ways to Cope with Them), Aile ve Toplum Eğitim-Kültür ve Araştırma Dergisi, 2007;11(3):99-108.

[2] Serin NB, Öztürk S. Anne-Babası Boşanmış 9-13 Yaşlarındaki Çocuklar İle Aynı Yaş Grubundaki Anne-Babası Boşanmamış Çocukların Benlik Saygısı ve Kaygı Düzeyleri (The Relationship Between The Self Esteem and The Anxiety Levels of Children Between The Age 9-13 Whose Parents had Divorced The Same Range of Whom are not Divorced), Ahi Evran Üniversitesi Kırşehir Eğitim Fakültesi Dergisi (KEFAD), 2007;2(8):117-128.

[3] Akyüz E. Boşanmanın Çocuk Üzerindeki Etkileri (Effects of Divorce on Children), http://dergiler.ankara.edu.tr/dergiler/40/500/ 5949.pdf. Erişim tarihi: 18 July 2014.

[4] Öndiger N. Boşanmanın Çocuk Üzerindeki Etkileri (Effects of Divorce on Children), Psikiyatride Güncel Yaklaşımlar, 2013; 5(2):140-161.

[5] Column P. Divorce and Children With Chronic Disorders: Diabetes as an Exemplar, Lipman T. H. (Edts), The Children's Hospital of Philadelphia, Philadelphia, 2013: 311-312. http://dx.doi.org/10.1016/j.pedn.2013.03.001.

[6] Uçan O. Boşanma Sürecinde Kriz Merkezine Başvuran Kadınların Retrospektif Olarak Değerlendirilmesi (Retrospective Evaluation of Women who Applied Crisis Center in Divorce Duration) Klinik Psikiyatri 2007;10:38-45, http://klinikpsikiyatri.org/system/files/journals/1/256.pdf. Erişim Tarihi: 20.07.2014.

[7] Alkaynak B. Çocuk ve Ergen Psikiyatrisi Temel Kitabı (Basic Book of Child and Adolescent Psychiatry), Boşanma ve Çocuk (Divorce and Children), Çocuk ve Gençlik Ruh Sağlığı Derneği Yayınları.

[8] Çivitçi A, Çivitçi N, Fiyakalı NC. Anne-Babası Boşanmış Olan Ergenlerde Yalnızlık ve Yaşam Doyumu (Adolescents with divorced parents Loneliness and Life Satisfaction), Kuram ve Uygulamada Eğitim Bilimleri, Pamukkale Üniversitesi Eğitim Fakültesi, Psikolojik Danışma ve Rehberlik Anabilim Dalı Öğretim Üyesi, Denizli Mustafa Kaynak Anadolu Lisesi Rehber Öğretmeni, Eğitim Danışmanlığı ve Araştırmaları İletişim Hizmetleri Tic. Ltd. Şti., 2009:493-525.

[9] Arifoğlu B, Richard NŞ, Razı G, Öz F. Çocuklar İçin Boşanmaya Uyum Envanteri Geçerlik ve Güvenirlik Çalışması, (The Child's Divorce Adjustment Inventory: A Study of Validity and Reliability), Çocuk ve Gençlik Ruh Sağlığı Dergisi, 2010;17:121-127.

[10] Çelen M. "Türkiye'de Boşanma Olgusu ve Boşanma Çeşitleri (Types of Divorce and Divorce Case in Turkey)", Ulusal Aile Sempozyumu-Sebep ve Sonuçlarıyla Boşanma Olgusu Sempozyumu (Sözel bildiri), Yuva Kurma ve Aileyi Koruma Derneği, Adana:10.04.2011.

[11] Geçikli E. Boşanma, Ebeveyn ve Çocuk (Divorce, Parents and Children), T.C. Lüleburgaz Kaymakamlığı Lüleburgaz İlçe Milli Eğitim Müdürlüğü, 2012. www.hukuksokagi.com

[12] http://hekimce.com/index.php?kiid=2888. Baby and Familie dergisi, Şubat 2006;02. Erişim Tarihi: 21.07.2014.

[13] Semerci ZB. Ergen Ruh Sağlığı (Aileler ve Ergenler için), (Adolescent Mental Health), İstanbul: Alfa Yayınları, 2007.

[14] Tunalı D. Anne ve Çocuk Dizisi 5 (Mother and Child Series) Çocuk Sağlığı Rehberi, Tunalı D.(Çvr Edts), Amerikan Tıp Birliği.

[15] Arifoğlu B, Öz F. Boşanmış Aile Çocuklarına Hemşirelik Yaklaşımı (Nursing Approach Toward Children with Divorced Parents), Hacettepe Üniversitesi Sağlık Bilimleri Fakültesi Hemşirelik Dergisi, 2008;76-84.

[16] Carpenito LJ. Handbook of Nursing Diagnosis. 7th Edition. Philadelphia, Newyork: Lippincott.Firdevs Erdemir (Çev. Edt). Hemşirelik Tanıları El Kitabı. İstanbul: Nobel Tıp Kitabevleri Ltd. Şti. ISBN: 975-420-020-3. 1999.

[17] Birol L. Hemşirelik Süreci (Nursing Process), 7. Baskı, İzmir: Etki Matbaacılık Yayıncılık; 2005.

Chapter 6

Chronic Health Conditions in Childhood and Adolescence and the Formation of Care and Support Networks

Camila Aloisio Alves

Additional information is available at the end of the chapter

http://dx.doi.org/10.5772/59060

1. Introduction

Addressing care and support networks issues in the chronic health conditions context for children and adolescents requires understanding chronicity within the contemporary scenario and its nuances, both as a trace of epidemiological transition and through experiences that emerge from dealing with illnesses.

Chronicity features the healthcare offered to patients as complex, since it requires specialized professional expertise, as well as the mastery of specific technologies and assistance techniques. Relationships established among professionals, patients and their families are quite intense and interactive, due to the need for continuous monitoring. At the same time, chronic patients need a sort of care which is not provided by specific actions from certain specialties only. It requires coordination among fields of knowledge and actions from different professionals and institutions.

According to the experience of patients and families, chronicity is complex because of all the repercussions it has on their lives. Experiencing pain, suffering, and distress facing diagnosis, treatment and rehabilitation are among the set of conditions that shape chronic disease frames in children and adolescents. Management of everyday life undergoes changes, and the search for appropriate treatment leads patients and their families to the establishment of an itinerary towards getting health services.

Care and support networks raise as key elements to healthcare practices applied to chronic children and adolescents, helping them withstanding the impact from such experiences and, at the same time, to be able to walk the paths to meet the necessary healthcare practices for their illness conditions. Chronic conditions demand a necessary care which needs to be structured in order to encourage exchanges among different individuals, institutions and social sectors. From the care and support network's perspective, the other one can be seen and understood *"as a living being in a state of interrelation and interdependence with all phenomena, which means enhancing pediatric practice"* [1, p.174].

Thus, the current chapter will address chronic health conditions in childhood and adolescence from a social anthropological perspective, therefore giving visibility to experiences emerging from clinical practices involving illnesses in order to be able to set the role played by care and support networks within this context.

2. Chronic health conditions

Brazil's demographic and epidemiological profile has undergone deep changes over the last century. In the early twentieth century, Brazil was a country characterized by high mortality rates caused by infectious and parasitic diseases. Due to the contribution of health and sanitation technologies, such as vaccination, hygiene, childcare and investments in health education, the country has seen its population grow and increase its life expectancy over the decades.

Chronic degenerative diseases have become more significant, prevalent and incident as an epidemiological feature of this change, even if concurrently with infectious and parasitic diseases in their epidemic or endemic form.

Chronic health conditions were gradually taking up space in service dynamics, professionals' trainings, health policies, pharmaceutical industry production, research and scientific studies. Such Brazilian profile, in line with other developed or developing countries, indiscriminately affects regions and social classes [2].

In the course of an individual's life, the emergence of a chronic health condition usually involves permanent changes in his/her usual routines, intrapersonal and interpersonal relationships, eating and physical habits, and the interaction with health services. Such changes can be explained by the need to introduce control, preventive and protective measures against the disease. People with chronic diseases need more supportive, planned and integrated healthcare. They are patients who need support from their communities and also need comprehensive policies for preventing or effectively managing chronic conditions. The optimal treatment for chronic conditions requires a new healthcare system model [2].

The new model indicated by the World Health Organization requires professionals able to establish an integrated and interdisciplinary care system as well as to create links among subjects, services and care levels.

With the emergence of chronic conditions, the Brazilian healthcare system faces illness profiles that require continuous attention, with measures aimed at both treating and managing the condition, as well as preventing it at different levels. The system bottleneck regards the worsening of the chronic conditions. Its impact is felt when clinical status worsens, thus increasing the demand for admission to ICU beds. The exacerbation of chronic conditions impacts on care provision costs and on the financial investment in medicines, supplies and technological resources to be used in treatments.

Chronic conditions impose a limit to health professionals due to the search for a resolutive care aiming at healing. Furthermore, chronic patients need more frequent and intense contact with professionals. It requires such professionals to develop dialogical and communicative skills that make patients feel welcome.

In this sense, chronicity brought into question the way services work and how health professionals interact in order to provide care. As chronicity happens, disciplinary separating among professional categories has become critical and requires an integration exercise based on dialogue and interdisciplinary attitudes.

3. Chronic health conditions in childhood and adolescence

Regarding child and adolescent health context, demographic and epidemiological transitions meet what was observed in the general population. It is characterized by the increase in overweight, childhood obesity, reduced malnutrition and reduced mortality rates among children at the age group from two months to five years.

The list of chronic conditions that affect children and adolescents is extensive. According to Castro and Piccinini [3, p. 624] they can be listed as follows: Organic chronic diseases (e.g.: cystic fibrosis, congenital heart diseases, chronic renal failure, biliary atresia, cirrhosis, cancer, hemophilia, AIDS); Physical impairments (e.g.: deformity or absence of a body limb, cleft lip and palate, visual and hearing impairment); Learning disabilities and neurological disorders (e.g.: epilepsy, cerebral palsy, attention deficit); Mental illness (e.g.: autism); and also Psychosomatic diseases (e.g.: asthma, obesity).

Technological and scientific contributions, in addition to control and prevention measures, have had a strong impact in this scenario. They allowed increasing survival rates of children who were born with or developed some of these pathologies.

The basis of these conditions articulates biological, psychological and/or cognitive aspects. Therefore, they seriously impact the lives of patients and their families enabling the development of limited functions or activities and affecting their social relationships when taking under account their dependence on medicines, medical technologies and special diets [4].

Chronicity experiences might begin early in pregnancy. Giving birth to a baby at risk may trigger a chronic condition already expected, felt and experienced throughout all pregnancy stages. A number of feelings such as fear, uncertainty, doubt, anger and guilt can be felt at each pregnancy month, thus requiring preparation procedures so the family can be ready for the labor.

A baby who shows some problem early in pregnancy, during labor or shortly after it is considered a baby at risk and such risk may trigger a chronic condition. Prenatal medical practices together with tests, investigations, monitoring procedures and counseling are extremely important to ensure good assistance [5].

Current technologies and proper prenatal assistance throughout pregnancy include being aware of the pregnancy evolution as well as of risks and possible outcomes, all based on diagnoses. Risks and/or chronic conditions in children are experienced from early pregnancy stages. It means that the arrival of these children can be prepared, although it is nonetheless distressing.

Experiencing chronic diseases in its core means facing the uncertainty of future life conditions that affect not just the medical approach, but and above all, the destiny of patients who, in many cases, see themselves as suppressed of the possibility of making long-term projects.

Giving birth to a baby diagnosed with some risk and/or chronic condition requires the presence of trained professionals and technologies capable of supporting life within the delivery room. The use of striking technologies within the chronic conditions context involves family and children during pregnancy, labor and throughout the child's life [5].

After such baby is born, he/she begins a bond building process different from that which happens with "normal" babies, those with no chronic conditions. It happens due to the need of taking the child away from the mother – the first stays in the ICU whereas the mother stays in the hospital room. "This is a difficult time, as well as it is to be discharged without being able to take the baby home" [6, p 24].

According to Braga and Morsch [7], getting into an ICU full of devices, sounds, tough situations, tubes, wires and requirements can be an experience surrounded by feelings such as fear and bewilderment, even for parents who were informed and prepared to face the birth of a child at risk.

Gradually, the family needs to know the world around the baby and how to communicate with the child, as well as to understand what is happening and how to recognize the baby's reactions.

According to Braga and Morsch [8], parents usually need a waiting period before they can begin to approach the child. Such period holds both the fear of losing the baby and the search for ways to establish parental relationship. Through this relationship built in the ICU environment, they begin to establish familiarity with and get aware of the care environment.

According to the authors, mothers have difficulties in expressing and developing their primary maternal concerns[1] because such concerns are mediated by another type of concern which is related to monitoring the child's health clinical evolution [7].

Thus, accessing, learning and mastering the knowledge and techniques which are common in the biomedical scenario are gradually learned and experienced by parents. These competencies

1 The primary maternal concern develops itself from the beginning of the pregnancy, becoming more intense in the final pregnancy period and after birth. It can last for months after the delivery. It is a mother's psychological state in which her sensitivity to the child becomes exacerbated [9].

and skills are incorporated and implemented in the course of the child's life, whether in hospital, either at home.

Children born with chronic conditions, and diagnosed in the very first moments of life, are assisted by Neonatology. If they survive, they are transferred to pediatric wards. The adaptation to everyday life, in face of a chronic condition, is implemented from the moment the child is transferred to the NICU. Professionals follow the child's health evolution and his/her possible needs of other services such as Intermediate Care Unit, Pediatric Surgery and Pediatrics.

Neonatal and pediatric patients living with a chronic condition since early age explore the world and develop their perceptions, emotions, learning and relationships through and despite their condition, knowing no other way to walk through life. In addition, just as the children, family members improve through experiencing hospital relationships and procedures, and by learning new ways of being mothers, fathers, brothers, grandfathers, grandmothers to chronic babies.

However, the onset of a chronic condition may occur during the development of the child and it can also lead to changes in both patients and families routines. From the very beginning of the investigation up to the confirmation of the clinical condition, children begin to adapt themselves to new circumstances and deal with suffering, possible limitations and with the fear of dying [10]. Cystic fibrosis is an example of this kind of situation, since it only shows its first symptoms later in the child's life.

The emergence of a chronic disease in adolescence causes a sudden interruption of "normal" life. The onset of chronicity in a teenager's life interferes in bonds built among peers and in important moments experienced with friends and family. Adolescence is strongly related to different discoveries (body, sexuality and forms of sociability), as well as to the construction of identity and dreams to be fulfilled in the adulthood. It is a time of discovery, growth, development and expansion of autonomy. When the chronic condition onsets, it causes gaps in this process and may trigger the cycle of feelings reported by Faulhaber[12]: anger at the news, depression in face of the symptoms and changes in routine, apathy in face of a life limited by the illness and hospital environments, and resignation towards an unchangeable condition.

Whether they are diagnosed at birth or later in life, chronic health conditions in children and adolescents are permeated by high institutional processes, the transferring of responsibilities among professionals, and the greater occupation of hospital areas by family members since part of the family life is moved to the hospitalization context.

Accordingly, hospitalization or even re-hospitalization are experiences marked by a double break: for the mothers, regarding the family routine; and for patients, regarding the familial and social scene, with changes in habits involving: attending school, being with a group of friends, going to parks and practicing sports [11].

These changes cause strange feelings towards the hospitalization experience which will be felt differently by patients and their families. References from children and adolescents life context are replaced by light colored walls, invasive procedures, medicines, machinery, new terms and words, and by pain and suffering, thus modifying patients' life routine [13].

In cases of children with chronic conditions, their relationship with the illness changes and new skills are learned by them. Many of them grow up dealing with life limiting situations and learning to incorporate the hospital space into their everyday life.

Taking into account that children with a chronic condition may become a chronic adult[14], it is essential considering that his/her growth will be linked to such care relationships. Therefore, it is necessary to overcome the developmental view that sees children as beings under formation and incomplete and who, therefore, need to follow cultural and educational standards in order to regulate and normalize their future as adults [15].

Castro's[15] theory of action emphasizes the importance of legitimating children and adolescents as individuals able to exercise their rights by their ability to act in and understand the world. This statement is not different from the aforementioned, since it takes chronic health conditions in children and adolescents under account because through each diagnosis there is a story of life to be lived, told and respected.

4. Chronic health conditions under anthropological and sociological perspectives

The care given to a chronic condition patient requires concerns about his/her life path. Different surveys and studies were developed aiming to understand such path. It allowed building a consistent knowledge framework about chronic health conditions in order to better address them.

Socio-anthropological studies provide key elements for understanding chronic conditions, since they focus on the illness experience and its consequences in the individuals' lives. Studying the socio-cultural dimension of chronic conditions is a task aimed at understanding a subject's life element that explains and represents the sociocultural and family context [16].

Socio-anthropological studies on chronic conditions emerged in the 70s. Since then, studies have sought, despite the range of diseases that compose such conditions, to make distinctions among them and to understand the experience of living with the disease [11].

Chronic conditions force patients to live a life with uncertain course of events. Such uncertainty affects both the patients who are managing their lives, and health professionals who use some resources in order to provide care[11].

Canesqui [16] conducted an extensive and thorough documentary study, given her 25 years (1980-2005) of anthropological research in international journals of reference in the area. The synthesis produced by the author revealed that chronic conditions point out aspects related to private and everyday life, routine breaks, managing the disease and life itself. She also emphasizes that the care provided to the patient is not limited to the hospital environment.

The experience of a chronic disease can be understood as socially constructed, being inserted in time and in the social and historical space. When faced by a chronic disease, everyday life's structure is transformed, changed, thus requiring subjects to mobilize resources from different orders so they can deal and cope with the disease, making their life trajectories being traced according to the possibilities and limitations imposed by the disease. It is an adjustment process with moments of accommodation, struggle and redefinition [16].

As the chronic disease evolves, it changes the patients' perceptions about themselves, the same way that it encourages the production of strategies for coping with it. Inevitably, the chronic disease causes the subject to be in touch with the possibilities of exercising some autonomy in life [16].

Living with the disease requires the subject to build strategies to deal with the different spheres of life, seeking re-adaptations that are able to establish a rhythm for the course of their lives [11].

In this sense, having or developing a chronic condition involves, according to the patients perspective, rebuilding their personal identity that is constantly shaped by the disease and its limitations. This reconstruction can be related to living with aesthetic changes, depending on technology, learning new body movements and adopting preventive measures [16].

In the set of studies on the subject, there is one developed by Goffman [17] which addresses stigma as an experience that may be related to having a chronic condition able to affect and deteriorate patient's identity. Regarding the identity of a chronic condition patient, Canesqui [16] points out the existence of two possible explanations. The first one emphasizes the strength of the community, with its rules represented as expectations and stereotypes expressed in personal experience conditioning. The second one has the opposite sense; it demonstrates that the individual's experience with the disease stimulates collective actions. According to the second line of thought, there are researches focused on the legitimacy of chronic conditions, such as backaches, arthritis and arthrosis, that are not valued or are not subject to constant suspicion, due to lack of etiologic evidence. Such studies focus on the subjects' pilgrimage through health services and their struggle against the way they are labeled.

Other than that, chronic conditions, when diagnosed inside the womb and/or at birth, mark the history of the child and his/her family, whether for the fact that they are not going to meet the expectations and dreams of a "normal" life, or for the need of re-adaptation in face of possible limitations and/or routine changes imposed by the condition itself.

The experience of a chronic condition is not limited to the patient. It also involves the family and health professionals. A Mexican study [18] investigated the perspectives of patients and health professionals (medical and non-medical) in face of chronic diseases. Results showed different aspects, demonstrating that the point of view on a particular experience (social role, life path, etc.) is related to the individuals' role within the social relationship context.

The patients highlighted the disease symptoms, the emotional manifestations in face of the challenges of living with pain, limitations permeated by health professional orientations (diet, medications, activities, procedures), and they also pinpointed aspects related to religiousness and spirituality as elements of support, strength and belief. Relatives were sometimes mentioned as supporting elements, or as conflict sources due to the difficulties of dealing with the patients' limitations regarding special care [18].

Non-medical professionals highlighted patients' emotional breakdown resulting from difficulties to deal with their conditions and physical problems arising from clinical worsening. They also underlined the economic and labor effects arising from the partial or total suspension of their labor activities. In addition, they mentioned the uncontrolled clinical state of health in face of the failure in following the doctor's requirements or the difficulty in having access to the necessary resources [18].

Finally, doctors prioritized the emotional manifestations, symptoms and organic signs, the effects from prescriptions that sometimes are followed, sometimes are not, the explanations of genetic background, featuring a more prescriptive relationship with the patients [18].

In this context, it is possible to understand that, during more than 30 years of socio-anthropological studies, the objects varied and results revealed different experiences from living with chronic diseases, placing subjects with chronic conditions in the center of both the analysis and the synthesis. Chronic conditions represent not only an epidemiological and demographic movement of a population's social dynamics and health, but they also refer to ways of experiencing life, existing in the world and establishing relationships.

5. Care and support networks

Due to the complexity imposed by chronic health conditions to children and adolescents, the development of a comprehensive caregiving system that articulates different specialties and integrates health services network is seen as necessary. The experience of chronicity in children and adolescents, besides affecting their life trajectories, involves the intense participation of family members accompanying them. The chronic condition requires continuous and long-term care which is, in general, provided and managed by family members. Family involvement comes with significant changes in family members' routines. Moving to a new house or switching and sometimes losing the job is likely due to the need of providing continuous care to the children.

Temporality in chronic conditions leads to exacerbation and stabilization periods. It requires families to take different measures in order to provide care. In stabilization times, the family's rhythm is driven to be reconfigured in order to deal with a new routine, which is marked by constant monitoring signs, symptoms, medication and nutrition management. On the other hand, in exacerbation times, the demand for health services is more intense.

Therefore, in addition to the technical aspects that characterize healthcare qualification, such as intensive, nutritional, respiratory and environmental cares, the support provided to family members is seen as a necessary element to the composition of a comprehensive care.

The comprehensive care for chronic health conditions in children and adolescents involves not only the use of hard technologies, such as equipment, medicines, medical examinations and procedures, but also soft technologies[2], such as welcoming families and a dialogic relationship that enables family members to be co-involved in and take co-responsibility for providing care to the children. All these elements ensure that caregiving for chronic health conditions in children and adolescents is complex and multifaceted, since it must be thought under a horizontal and humanized perspective.

Families should be considered as primary caregiving units, systems of belonging that value the bond and ties of solidarity, trust and donation, to which resources must converge, relying on the organization of practices from networks and links [20, 21].

The way children and families face chronic disease is associated with family organization and interaction factors. The support from the family and social ties, the family support networks as well as patients' protection networks serve as a social fabric that which allows improving the management of experienced situations. The construction of support networks among family members and friends can happen during the process of looking for care and support. Building such links helps ensuring patients' well-being [11, 22].

In the context of chronic conditions, the experience lived by family and friends who are united by bonds and ties, in facing adverse situations and reconfiguring their life routines, is studied by authors who address therapeutic itineraries and care trajectories [20, 21, 23, 24].

The formation and structuring of networks from links and bonds established among family members and friends are not fixed. They can change according to the momentary needs, showing reticular and individual movements that happen within and between networks [20].

The formation of networks in the context of chronic health conditions in children and adolescents is a feature that should be considered as an integral part of caregiving. For many families, the sense of belonging to a network of friends, families, neighbors and professionals represents a great difference in their life trajectories. Through such networks, one can access services, share experiences and build knowledge about the experienced problem.

Care and support networks can be woven and built in different spaces where patients and their families seek for care and treatment. There are contact points for networks conformation among friends and family community, as well as among and within health services.

In hospitalization contexts, as children and adolescents with chronic conditions show higher average length of permanence in hospitals and accompanying people have their presence guaranteed by law throughout the hospitalization process, family members get to know and learn about the logic of hospital functioning and about procedures and clinical parameters. The intensity of such experience puts accompanying people of different patients in contact, so they are bonded by the common experience of being chronic children caregivers.

A common identity is built among family members, and through it, they are able to share the burden of hospitalization. It creates opportunities for exchanging experiences, sharing knowledge, trust and solidarity thus contributing for the family to feel safe. Many times, the

---

2 According to contemporary authors, such as Merhy et al. [19, p. 121], the work in health services is considered as alive, because its object is not fully structured and its actions are configured as intervention processes in action, working through relationships, subjectivities confluence, in addition to the structured technological knowledge. The used technologies can be considered as "soft, soft-hard and hard". The first one relates to the production of bonding, welcoming, autonomy and management; the second one refers to the structured knowledge in different specialties, and the last one relates to the technologies applied to the field.

absence of a mother-who needs to go home to change clothes and take care of other children-is feasible because another mother, who accompanies her child in the next bed, makes herself available to take care of the child during maternal absence.

Therefore, the use of resources such as family groups is essential to the trajectory of chronic children and adolescents caregivers. In groups composed of family members, individuals who experience adverse situations are able to share common experiences since they are gathered by their children conditions. It allows creating bonds and ties, even if temporarily, which are strong in their ability to add value to therapeutic itineraries and caregiving trajectories [20, 21, 23, 24].

Strategies to support relatives and patients are also found in hospital environment and they work as networks of affection, care, support and assertion to the individual's identity beyond the pathology. Recreational activities, open visits for siblings and grandparents, hospital classes and reading programs are among such strategies.

Recreational activities should compose the scene of support networks for patients, because playful activities used as a therapeutic resource deals with social, cultural and psychological aspects. Through playful activities, experiences related to the hospital environment, such as discomfort caused by procedures, pain and fear find another communication channel. Furthermore, affection bonds and relationships are exchanged through the contact with professionals who propose such activities.

Playing is an activity that favors the creation of alliances and interactions among patients, their families and professionals, allowing the construction of a new social network and helping to decrease the sense of isolation and loneliness caused by hospitalization [25]. Regarding the child/accompanying person relationship, playing can also rebuild fragmented ties derived from the family chaos caused by the disease [26].

Including "playing" in hospitalization contexts both respects the uniqueness of each child and serves as a means of expressing their pain and their joy. Playing helps democratically transforming the hospital space by valorizing the individual's experiences and autonomy exercises [13].

In addition to recognizing children and adolescents as individuals, hospital classes serve as elements working on cognitive and skills development. Besides contributing to the education of hospitalized children and adolescents, hospital classes represent a care technology by contributing to their quality of life. This is an element of social inclusion, which recognizes patients as individuals with rights that must be preserved [27]. Such classes recognize the dignity of patients, which should be respected as well as their chronic condition. Reading programs working through the playful aspect of reading to babies, children, adolescents and their families follow the same direction. Such resources give rise to other ways of understanding the patients beyond their clinical condition, encouraging playfulness and joy.

The introduction of siblings' visits to the hospital context is another important aspect. This is a strategy that helps the sibling at home to get closer to the new family member. For mothers, it is a means of integrating the family, reducing concerns, enabling rapprochements and conversations that can modulate the experience for everyone involved in the process.

http://dx.doi.org/10.5772/59060

According to Morsch and Braga [28], the siblings' visit is a time of family integration. Given children's spontaneity, questions, new meanings, gestures and behaviors emerge from the siblings gathering, allowing possible barriers between the hospitalized baby and his/her relatives to be broken.

According to the American Academy of Pediatrics and the Ministry of Health in Brazil through the Children's Program, the siblings visit practice is stimulated due to its results focused on healthcare humanization, favoring bonds of affection and links among family members and the hospitalized child. However, the entry of siblings should always be accompanied by a conversation with the professionals in charge in order to clear out doubts regarding how to proceed in such moments [28].

Authors [28] reported the benefits identified in meetings that happen during the hospitalization of children and adolescents: they provide a reduction in children complaints in face of an unknown situation and, in small children, improvements can be observed in possible associated symptoms, such as: sleep, eating, and defecation disorders. Closeness among siblings helps building a sense of belonging.

Similarly, the presence of grandparents in the hospitalization context has been studied as a feature that allows the development of an extended mothering[3], favoring the support for parents who usually get emotionally worn by the child's hospitalization. Since grandparents did not undergo the psychological transformation of pregnancy, childbirth and puerperium, they become key figures to offer more support [8].

The possibility of a grandmother to be present during her grandchild's hospitalization favors sharing experiences with someone the mother trusts. As for the baby, according to Braga and Morsch [8] (p. 82), *"we can make him/her [the child or baby] feel welcome to the world, to the extent that he/she will have more interlocutors to expand his/her communication skills."*

The great potential of networks formed within chronic conditions care environment is to recognize individuals and their needs, and through such recognition, produce subjectivities born from more dialogue interactions among professionals, caregivers and patients. It contributes, therefore, to rescue the autonomy of individuals involved with caregiving and of those who need it [29].

By the strategies described in the preceding paragraphs, it is possible to see the inclusion of children and adolescents as individuals with rights, as well as the recognition and establishment of affection bonds and support among individuals (professionals and family) who work with caregiving to chronic children and adolescents. Ties and bonds built through such strategies help coping with the pain and anguish derived from chronicity and contributes to sharing strategies and solutions related to them.

Therefore, professionals can also be individuals who contribute to the construction of a care network, by developing comprehensive care strategies, articulating sectors and services as well as by sharing information with family members.

---

3 The term extended mothering refers to the inclusion of individuals or a group of family members in contexts in which a caretaker is absent. They can support, participate and follow the pregnancy and the early baby care [7].

The role of professionals in this context is crucial and it can go beyond the institutions' walls, facilitating the articulation among services during the search for specialized references. Building a horizontal relationship with family members and a detailed knowledge of each case can assist patient and family mobilization through the health network. Favoring the conformation of such ties and the users path through the network by accessing other health care networks is a movement called by Fontes [30, p.124] as "social relay". Through "social relay", it is possible to build "networks of networks", which helps empowering the family in face of the child's chronicity.

In the study by Alves, Oliveira and Mourão [31], empowerment was analyzed according the patients, families and professionals involved in caregiving to chronic mental health conditions. As for patients and their families, empowerment comes from the experience acquired through knowledge, information and qualification on the disease. Such a concept makes sense when individuals are able to relate, talk and have more freedom to live, speak, participate and exchange experiences. As for professionals, empowerment is built by favoring patients' better understanding of their disease and of the world they live in, as well as by contributing to the exercise of their autonomy.

However, in Brazil, when people speak about networks outside hospital walls, the scenario seems to be fragile, still under construction and with little dialogue process among institutions, whether because of the almost lack of services and support actions, or because professionals do not know where and who to look for. Support networks conformation is still very limited to some professionals' initiatives in seeking for access and articulating demands to the existing services in the territories. Such scenario weakens the establishment of bonds and caregiving which could strengthen the integration among services and care levels.

In the Brazilian context of child health care, there is the "Child-Health Network". Such network was launched in the 90s and was formed by voluntary associations that recognized each other and organized themselves aiming to provide support and social monitoring to chronic children and adolescents and to their families. Moreira [32], when analyzing the associative construction based on the willingness and solidarity found in such arrangements, highlights the donation system born from it, since it is possible to recognize the role of reciprocity in relationships. Reciprocity operates in the donation process on the part of those seeking to help and of those who receive such help. The association mediates relationships and monitors benefited families by introducing sociability mechanisms among individuals. Thus, it operates on a horizontal field of relationships towards a common project, opening itself for cultivating personal relationships [32].

In order to provide a comprehensive care for children and adolescents with chronic health conditions, it is necessary to integrate services and care levels. Professionals' synergy efforts can be increased through such integration.

Network conformations, inside or outside of the services, can be understood as a means to produce association and interaction among individuals. Social capital and symbolic exchanges circulate through social networks in which professionals help each other and assist users, allowing donation to be enabled by the giving, receiving and reciprocating circuit [33].

From the public health policies perspective, in recent years in Brazil, the investment in care network conformations has been growing in view of the impact of chronic health conditions prevalence and incidence. Mendes [34] indicates the prospect of care networks articulated by Primary Health Care as a proposition for rethinking the chronic conditions care model. The main aspect in such proposition is to overcome the health system fragmentation to the extent that, through PHC, it would work in coordination with other care levels, exceeding the hierarchical pyramid vertical logic of complexity levels.

Health care networks are "polyarchic organizations of health care services linked by a single mission, common goals and by a cooperative and interdependent action. They allow a specific population to be provided with a comprehensive and continuous support, which is coordinated by Primary Health Care " [34, p. 2300]. Based on such understanding and conformation, networks would establish ways of providing a more resolutive assistance to patients. It is important to emphasize that the model seeks to articulate services and provide continuous care so that the user is the center of a line of conduct. It is also important that the actions can be articulated in different levels. In addition, health professionals should not be the ones exclusively in charge of the care, since such charge should be shared among all subjects.

WHO [2] highlights that chronic conditions imply a paradigm shift not only in performing, but also in organizing and managing health activities and services in order to allow an alignment of sector policies, by emphasizing prevention based on scientific evidences and developing an articulated and integrated system focused on the patient, his/her family and community.

The requirements placed by WHO [2] and Mendes [34] concern the demands imposed by chronic conditions to health services due to the gap existing in the historically constructed health care model. However, one of the central aspects related to chronicity is at the heart of this issue: the prolongation of an incurable condition that changes the individual's life routine and that occupies the center of all social relationships [11].

The profile of a demand arising from chronic conditions concerns a kind of care that is not extinguished by the time the patient is discharged. Providing a continuous care is essential, but the unpreparedness of the other network edges results in the non-inclusion of patients in other care levels, because there are no pacts or flows to guide both professionals and users.

According to Sousa, Erdmann and Mochel [35] the comprehensive care provided to chronic children and adolescents finds little or no assistance structure to fit the demands beyond hospital walls. Similarly, there is no effective reference and counterreference system for different the care levels.

Caring for chronic conditions requires not only academic and human training and investments focused on the hospitalization process, but also the management of levels, processes and flows that compose the health system.

Support networks are not just resources to be accessed but, above all, they are means of enhancing care, indicators that measure how much the formation of bonds and support is necessary to caregivers' trajectory: professionals and family. Undoubtedly, networks represent elements that point to health actions verticality failures and to the inevitable articulation and integration path among services and subjects.

According to Moreira and Goldani [14, p. 322], the current demands and new knowledge are shaping "new pediatrics" in which hospital-centered models are not efficient because they require greater articulation among services and care levels.

It is understood that, regarding support networks for chronic patients, there are stronger and weaker links. Some of them have greater chances of being developed and others are in an institutional radius of limited action sphere, such as family context issues. However, the more difficult the access is to networks, the greater the chance for professionals to feel frustrated in their work, since their action towards the child is limited, once they can only perform within their medical specialty.

Caring for chronic children and adolescents requires us to be able to look, understand and act in a comprehensive manner, which can only be achieved if there is a field of possibilities for exchanging, sharing as well as for establishing horizontality in services and among social actors.

As for a schematic approach, the discussion and reflection highlighted above and those that surround the Brazilian health policies scenario are shown in the Table 1. below:

Health System				
Levels of care	Primary care	Secondary care	Tertiary care	Quatarenary care
Services	Family health Homecare Core support to family health	Specialized health centers, polyclinics	Hospitals and reference centers	
Care and support activities	Makes the conection with the family, longitudinal follow-up of cases, articulates local services for support, assists in the integration of chronic children and adolescents back into society through intersectoral action, supports parents in caregiving	Diagnosis exam support, between appointments, consultations with specialists	Family groups/ Sibling visits. Hospital classes/ Recreational activities/ reading programs	
Areas and support services	Diagnostic support services/ Pharmaceutical care/ Emergency care			

Table 1. Organizing the health system, levels of attention and services to help chronic children and adolescents, according to the Brazilian experience:

The health system can be organized into attention levels (primary, secondary, tertiary and quaternary) that present services able to develop the actions of their competence. The study focused in promotion, prevention and assistance in the primary health attention. Brazil stands out for its family health strategies, the family health support and homecare; all of them comprised by services that set straight contact with families in order to give follow up on the cases. They articulate the local support services and help integrating chronic children and adolescents back into society through inter-sectorial actions as well as they give support to parents on caregiving.

The secondary level regards to services and procedures that aim at giving support to primary care, especially for chronic patients' caregiving, diagnosis exams support, inter-consultations and specialized consultations. Thus, it minimizes visits at the hospital to less complex activities and helps preventing complications and new hospital admissions.

Hospitals and reference services that can develop support activities and care to chronic children and adolescents and to their families, providing them with group ludic activities, visits from grandparents and siblings, besides activities focused on the pedagogical development such as classes and reading programs are found in the tertiary and quaternary levels.

Patients and their families must be in the center of the concerns not just from the health area but from all the areas involved with taking care of these individuals (education, social assistance, support associations, among others). According to the demands from the scenario of illnesses in chronic children and adolescents, effective answers result from the inter-section of different society sectors.

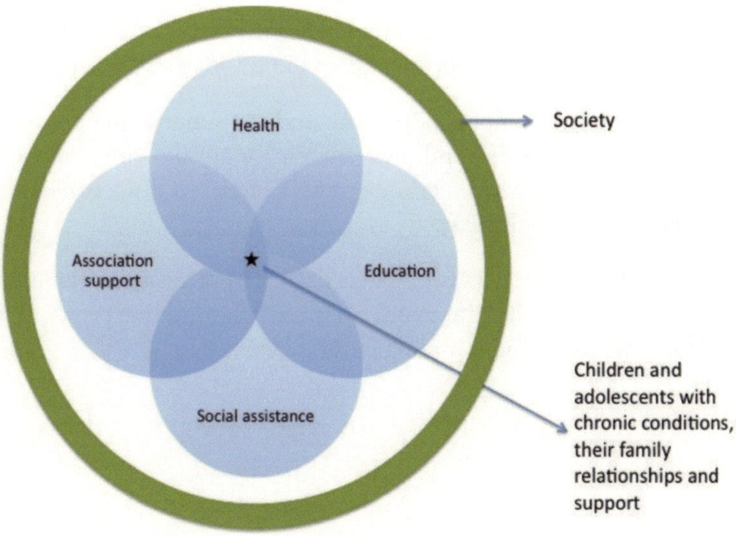

Figure 1. Picture of the articulation among society sectors focused on the care to children and adolescents with chronic conditions:

6. Final consideration

The contemporary health scenario has shown that chronic health conditions in children and adolescents do not refer to pathologies that are segregated to few groups of patients. These are health problems that cause serious effects on the lives of patients and their families, and that reorganize health services and professional practice, in general, affecting all society. Thus, they are conditions requiring the execution of a comprehensive care built by health, education and social assistance intersectorial fields.

Sociological and anthropological studies have shown that experiencing a chronic disease affects the lives of both the individuals and their family members, marking family routine management as well as patient's identity construction.

Chronic health conditions in children and adolescents should be understood beyond a demographic and epidemiological transition feature. They do not represent the end of a life, but an opening to other ways of being together in care encounters. Chronicity is a condition that can potentially create and reinvent ways of life and health. New meetings happen and, therefore, new bonds and forms of sociability and association can be built.

By understanding that chronic health conditions in children and adolescents represent different diseases which require multiple investments, promoting care and support networks helps generating greater integration among individuals, institutions and care levels.

Therefore, in this scenario, networks formation is multifactorial and multifaceted. It involves relationships among professionals, patients and their family members in whatever care context. Likewise, it requires institutional articulations which are both internal to the services that serve children and adolescents, and external, when involving other health system sectors. This set of links and bonds helps healthcare system to find solutions born from joint efforts.

The production of horizontality among individuals and institutions can generate a much more intense and rich field for knowledge and expertise exchange, allowing patients to be understood in a much more comprehensive and integrated manner. It also enables creating a kind of action that is, in fact, communicative.

In order to do so, it is necessary to revisit models used for professional training, services and health system organization so that the network perspective is a guiding principle in the exercise of horizontal actions and interactions among individuals.

Author details

Camila Aloisio Alves

Address all correspondence to: camila.aloisioalves@gmail.com

Fernandes Figueira Institute (IFF/Fiocruz) and Petrópolis Medical School, Brazil

References

[1] Santa Roza, E. Um desafio às regras do jogo: o brincar como proposta de redefinição da criança hospitalizada. In: Santa Roza, E.; Reis, E. S. (orgs) Da análise na infância ao infantil na análise. Rio de Janeiro: Contra Capa Livraria, 1997, pp. 161-187.

[2] World Health Organization. Cuidados inovadores para condições crônicas: componentes estruturais de ação: relatório mundial. Brasília. 2003

[3] Castro, E. K., Piccinini, C. A. Implications of Physical Chronic Disease in Childhood to Family Relationships: Some Theoretical Questions. Psicologia: Reflexão e Crítica, 2002, 15 (3) pp. 625-635.

[4] Silva, M. G. N. Chronic childhood: concept, prevalence and emotional repercussions. Revista de Pediatria do Ceará, 2001, 2 (2) pp. 29-32.

[5] Moreira, MEL.; Bomfim, OL.; Llerena Jr, J. Esperando um bebê de risco. In: Moreira, MEL.; Braga, NM.; Morsch, DS. Quando a vida começa diferente: o bebê e sua família na UTI neonatal. Rio de Janeiro: Editora Fiocruz, 2003, p. 15-22.

[6] Moreira, M.E.L.; Bomfim, O.L. Um nascimento diferente. In: Moreira, MEL.; Braga, NM.; Morsch, DS. Quando a vida começa diferente: o bebê e sua família na UTI neonatal. Rio de Janeiro: Editora Fiocruz, 2003, pp. 23-28.

[7] Braga, N.M.; Morsch, D.S. Os primeiros dias da UTI. In: Moreira, MEL.; Braga, NM.; Morsch, DS. Quando a vida começa diferente: o bebê e sua família na UTI neonatal. Rio de Janeiro: Editora Fiocruz, 2003, pp. 51-68.

[8] Braga N.M.; Morsch, D.S. Maternagem ampliada. In: Moreira, MEL.; Braga, NM.; Morsch, DS. Quando a vida começa diferente: o bebê e sua família na UTI neonatal. Rio de Janeiro: Editora Fiocruz, 2003, p. 81-98.

[9] Piccinini, C. A. A preocupação materna primária em mães de bebês nascidos pré-termo. Dissertação de mestrado. Porto Alegre. Universidade Federal do Rio Grande do Sul. Instituto de Psicologia. Curso de Pós-Graduação em Psicologia. 2009

[10] Pierre, A.; Kaufmann, A.; Waissman, R. Vivre une maladie grave: analyse d'une situations de crise. Revue Française de Sociologie, 1991, 32 (4) pp. 652-655.

[11] Adam, P. ; Herlizch, C. Sociologia da doença e da medicina. 1a. São Paulo: Edição EDUCS. 2001.

[12] Faulhaber, M. C. B. Enfermaria e o Adolescente. Disponível em: http://www.soperj.org.br/novo/publicacao_detalhes.asp?s=Publica%E7%F5es%20dos%20Comit%EAs&id=216. (acessado em julho, 2014).

[13] Mitre R.M.A. O Brincar no Processo de Humanização da Produção de Cuidados Pediátricos. In: Humanização dos cuidados em saúde: conceitos, dilemas e práticas. Deslandes, S.F. (org). Rio de Janeiro: Ed. Fiocruz. 2006, pp. 283-300.

[14] Moreira M.E.L. & Goldani M.Z. Child is the father of man: new challenges for child health. Ciência e Saúde Coletiva, 2010, 15 (2) pp. 321-327.

[15] Castro LR. Da invisibilidade à ação: crianças e jovens na construção da cultura. In: Crianças e Jovens na construção da cultura. p.19-46. Rio de Janeiro: Nau Editora – FAPERJ, 2001.

[16] Canesqui AM. Estudos Socioantropológicos Sobre os Adoecidos Crônicos. In: Olhares Socioantropológicos sobre os adoecidos crônicos. Canesqui AM (org) São Paulo: HUCITEC/FAPESP. 2007, pp.9-49.

[17] Goffman. I. Estigma – Notas sobre a Manipulação da Identidade Deteriorada. Rio de Janeiro: Editora Guanabara, 4a. Edição. 2004

[18] Mercado-Martinez; Hernandez-Hibarra. Chronic illness from the perspective of patients and health professionals: a qualitative study in México. Cad. Saúde Pública, 2007, 23 (9) pp. 2178-2186.

[19] Merhy EE. Em busca do tempo perdido: a micropolítica do trabalho vivo. In: Merhy EE., Onocko R R. (orgs). Agir em saúde: um desafio para o público. São Paulo: Hucitec, 2007, pp. 71-112.

[20] Santos de Araújo, l. F., Bellato, R., Hiller, M. Itinerário terapêutico e redes para o cuidado na condição crônica: algumas experiências. In: Pinheiro, R., Martins, P.H. N. Avaliação em Saúde na perspectiva do usuário: abordagem multicêntrica. Rio de Janeiro, Recife e São Paulo: CEPESC/IMS-UERJ; Editora Universitária UFPE; ABRASCO, 2009, pp. 203-216.

[21] Lopes, A. F. C., Walty, C. M. R. F., Duarte, E. D., Dittz, E. S., Lopes, T. C. Práticas de integralidade e as redes sociais: possibilidades avaliativas para a construção da cidadania de famílias de crianças em condições crônicas. In: Pinheiro, R., Matrins, P.H. N. Avaliação em Saúde na perspectiva do usuário: abordagem multicêntrica. Rio de Janeiro, Recife e São Paulo: CEPESC/IMS-UERJ; Editora Universitária UFPE; ABRASCO, 2009, pp. 217-228.

[22] Viana, V., Barbosa M.C.; Guimarães, J. Chronic disease in children familiar factors and quality of life. Psicologia, Saúde e Doenças, 2007, 8 (1) pp. 117-127.

[23] Bellato, R., Santos de Araújo, L.F., Faria, A.P.S., Correa da Costa, A. L., Maruyama, S. A. T. Itinerário terapêutico de famílias e redes para o cuidado na condição crônica: alguns pressupostos. In: Pinheiro, R., Martins, P.H. N. Avaliação em Saúde na perspectiva do usuário: abordagem multicêntrica. CEPESC/IMS-UERJ; Editora Universitária UFPE; ABRASCO, 2009, pp. 187-194.

[24] Costa, A. L. R. C., Figueiredo, D. L. B., Medeiros, L. H. L., Mattos, M., Maruyama, S. A. T. O percurso na construção de itinerários terapêuticos de famílias e redes para o cuidado. In: Pinheiro, R., Matrins, P.H. N. Avaliação em Saúde na perspectiva do usuário: abordagem multicêntrica. Rio de Janeiro, Recife e São PauloCEPESC/IMS-UERJ; Editora Universitária UFPE; ABRASCO, 2009, pp. 195-202.

[25] Mitre, R. Brincando para viver: Um estudo sobre a relação entre a criança gravemente adoecida e hospitalizada e o brincar,. Dissertação de mestrado, Rio de Janeiro: Instituto Fernandes Figueira, Fundação Oswaldo Cruz. 2000.

[26] Mitre, R.; Gomes, R. The play promotion in the context of childhood hospitalization as a health procedure. Ciência e Saúde Coletiva, 2004, 9 (1) pp. 147-154.

[27] Holanda, ER.; Collet, N. The difficulties of educating children with chronic illness in the hospital context. Rev Esc Enferm, 2011, 45 (2) 381-389.

[28] Morsch, D.S.; Braga, N.M. Os irmãos do bebê. In: Moreira, MEL.; Braga, NM.; Morsch, DS. Quando a vida começa diferente: o bebê e sua família na UTI neonatal. Rio de Janeiro: Editora Fiocruz, 2003, pp. 97-106.

[29] Duarte, MCS; Moreira, MCN. Autonomy and care in pediatric intensive care: the paradoxes of practice. Interface, 2011, 15 (38); pp.687-700.

[30] Fontes, B.A.S.M. Sobre trajetórias de sociabilidade: a ideia de rede de saúde comunitária. In: Martins, PH; Fontes, B. Redes sociais e saúde: novas possibilidade teóricas. Recife: Editora Universitária da UFPE. 2004, pp.121-139.

[31] Alves, T.C., Oliveira, W.F., Vasconcelos, EM. The viewpoint of users, families and professionals about empowerment in mental health. Physis Revista de Saúde Coletiva, 2013, 23 (1) 51-71.

[32] Moreira, M.C.N. Dádiva, reciprocidade e associação em rede na área da saúde: uma perspectiva sócio-antropológica. In: Martins, PH; Campos, RBC (org) Polifonia do dom. Recife: Editora Universitária da UFPE, 2006, pp.285-310.

[33] Moreira, M.C.N. Dádiva e rede na saúde: circuitos de troca e construção de estratégias de cuidado. In: Pineiro, R.; Mattos, RA. (Org.) Razões públicas para a integralidade em saúde: o cuidado como valor. Rio de Janeiro: CEPESC – IMS – ABRASCO, 2007, pp.301-316

[34] Mendes, EV. Health care networks. Ciência e Saúde Coletiva, 2010; 15 (5) 2297-2305.

[35] Sousa F.G.M, Erdmann A.L., Mochel E.G. Limiting conditions for intregal care for a child in brazilian primary health care. Texto Contexto Enferm, 2011; 20 (no. Esp) 263-71.

Section 4

Pediatric Surgery

Chapter 7

Dilemma in Teenager Varicocele

Hosni Khairy Salem

Additional information is available at the end of the chapter

http://dx.doi.org/10.5772/59314

1. Introduction

There is no subject that is more controversial in the area of male infertility than varicocele. Varicocele is the most common identifiable cause of male infertility. It can develop during puberty and thus affect the testicular growth and function. The incidence of varicocele in the adolescents is about 15 percent worldwide. Varicocele is associated with a time-dependent growth arrest in adolescents. There is a clear association between varicocele, infertility, and testicular growth arrest. It is also known that varicocelectomy can reverse growth arrest in adolescents. Considerable debate regarding the etiology and effects of adolescence varicoceles has appeared in the literature. This knowledge has raised the question of how best to manage adolescents with varicocele.

The chapter will discuss the following items:

a. The prevalence of adolescence varicocele.

b. Regional differences of adolescence varicocele.

c. Pathophysiology.

d. Anatomy.

e. The risk factors for the development of varicocele among boys.

f. Presentations.

g. The relations between the adolescent varicocele and puberty.

h. Evidence from controlled studies against varicocelectomy and the reports supporting varicocelectomy.

i. Bilaterality.

j. Whom we should repair.

k. Choice of repair.

2. The prevalence of adolescence varicocele

Varicocele means tortuosity and dilatation of the pampiniform plexus of veins inside the spermatic cord; it has been linked to infertility since 1955.

Varicocele is the most common identifiable cause of male infertility. It can develop during puberty and thus affect the testicular growth and function [1].

Varicocele affects 15-20% of adult men, 40% of adult men with primary infertility, 80% of men with secondary infertility, and 15 % of adolescents [2].

The incidence in older boys varies between 12.4% and 17.8% with an average of 14.2% [3].

This prevalence varies in different geographical areas.

In Balkan Peninsula, among Greece adolescents, the prevalence is only 3% among 3047 school boys. While the prevalence in Bulgarian boy's reaches 7.9% for the age group 10 to 19 years. Higher prevalence was detected in Turkish population reaching 11.02% in the age group 11 to 19 years old. [4-6].

3. Regional differences of adolescence varicocele

Kumanov et al in a prospective study evaluated 6200 boys aged 0 to 19 years from 5 regions in Bulgaria for the presence of varicocele. The icidence in whole group was found to be 4.1%, this icidence increases to 7.9% for the age group above 10 years old. The prevalence of varicocele demonstrated clear regional differences, the incidence of the disease increased rapidly during mid puberty [7].

The prevalence of varicocele was highest in the areas of Sofia and Varna, which are the largest cities in Bulgaria and was lowest in Vratza and Blagoevgrad which are the smallest towns in Bulgaria. The authors attributed the differences to be multifactorial, including enviromental factors and life style factors (physical development, food intake) [7].

4. Pathophysiology

In WHO study in 1992, including 9083 patient at 34 centers in 24 countries, it was proved that varicocele is classically associated with infertility and impaired testicular function [8].

Varicocele disrupts the groth and function of the testis with ultimate effect on fertility, many theoris have been suggested but none of them proved to be the ideal theory [9].

Hypothesis concerning the harmful effect of varicocele include; increase in the scrotal/ testicular temperature, elevation in the serum gonadotrophins level, increase in the venous pressure, accumulation of toxins, hypoxia and hormonal imbalance [10, 11].

5. Anatomy

Paduch and Skoog in 2001 suggested four theories to explain why the left sided varicocele is more predominat more than the right side. These theories include, nutcraker effect on left renal vein, increasing the blood supply to the testis at puberty exceeding the venous capacity, incomptent valves in the venous system, and high levels of nitric oxide in the pampiniform plexus of veins [3]. On the otherhand,Raman et al in 2005 suggested genetic susceptibility as a precipitating factor, considering that half of the first degree relatives and more than two third of the brothers of the patients with varicocele, also had clinical varicocele [4].

6. The risk factors for the development of varicocele among boys

It was found that the incidence of varicocele is related to some anthropometric and somatometric parameters [12-14]. Some studies discussed the protective role of higher BMI and/or weight on the development of varicocele [12-14]. Others discussed the negative influence of height [15, 16].

Obesity and high BMI may be correlated with increased adipose tissue in the spermatic cord which may lead to decrease in the detection of varicocele by examination [12-14].

In Kumanov et al study, the age of the boys, penile length, penile circumference, and height of the children, were positively related to the development of varicocele. The dark eye color also increased the risk for the anomaly. No relationship was found with hair color. In multivariate analysis, development of varicocele correlated negatively (predictive role) with the weight and BMI but correlated positively (protective role) with penile measurements (length, circumference) in addition to the height of the patients. The predictive role of the height was only evident in the first Tanner stages only with significant differences between the three stages seperately if compared with each others [7].

Tight clothing, constipation, wearing a truss, and presence of a tumor may be also a risk factor. Atheletes have high incidence of varicocele, spermatogenesis will be more affected in those sport-men with varicocele if the did vigorous physical activity [17, 18].

7. Presentations

Usually the presentation of varicocele in adolescents is asymptomatic, sometimes the patient presented by scrotal mass described as a bag of worms or testicular discomfort in the form of heaviness, dull aching pain on standing for long times. Not infrequently the presentation is small testicle if associated testicular hypotrophy occurred. Usually the diagnosis is made at routine hospital examination or as a prerequisite examination for employment or before engaging in a military service [19-23]..

8. The relations between the adolescent varicocele and puberty

With rapid linear growth spurt in adolescence at puberty, the nutcracker effect will become more evident with consequently increase in the hydrostatic pressure in the left testicular venous plexus [7, 10]. Moreover, the accelerated pubertal development with growth spurt and increased androgen secretion, in addition vasoactive compounds like inducible nitric oxide were suggested to play a role indevelopment of varicocele in the early stages of puberty. These vasoactive compounds were over expressed in the tesis and in the penile vaculature of patients with varicocele in the early stages of puberty [24].

Also, Sawczuk et al postulated that the increase in the arterial supply of the testis at puberty beyond the venous capacity may unmask an underlying hidden varicocele [25].

On the otherhand, Kumanov et al postulated that the rapid marked changes in the penile measurements and heights at puberty reflects endocrine and paracrine growth factors imbalance that act as a predisposing factor for the development of varicocele in genetically susceptible patients [7].

Testosterone is responsible for the adolescent secondary sexual characters (increase in the muscle mass, muscle tone, body hair, and level of sexual interest). Varicocele can damage the cells that make testosterone and lead to decrease over all testosterone level which may affect the adolescents in the mean time or in the future [26].

9. Evidence from controlled studies against varicocelectomy and the reports supporting varicocelectomy

In 1987, Kass and Belman found that 80% of boys with left varicocele with ipsilateral hypotrophy, exhibited catch up growth following varicocelectomy [27]..

10 years later, Sigman and Jarrow reported that a combination of varicocele and ipsilateral asymmetry was associated with higher incidence of abnormal semen parameters in a time dependent manner, this mean that varicocele is a progressive disease[28].

This opens the door for prophylactic varicocelectomy in adolescents in cases of ipsilateral asymmetry, hoping to prevent infertility when become older.

Okuyama et al reported on 24 boys who underwent varicocelectomy,67% of whom had initial left hypotrophy (group I) and 16 boys followed conservatively without surgery,50% of whom had initial left hypotrophy (group II). On follow up, 24% of group I have ipsilateral hypotrophy versus 75% in group II [29]..

When varicocele started early in adolescents, the damage to the germ cells as well as testicular atrophy will be greater [30-32]..

Repair of varicocele in adolescents reverse the testicular growth arrest and associated with catch up growth within one year of treatment, this mean that early detection and treatment of varicocele in adolescents is a preventive measure a against infertility [33].

The grade of varicocele has no relation to the testicular tissue damage, semen parameters preoperatively or improvement of the semen parameters postoperatively. Even sub clinical varicocele in adolescents may have significant effect on the testicular parenchyma and semen parameters [34-37].

The currently agreement indication for surgical repair of varicocele in adolescents include; testicular asymmetry more than 20% and persisted for more than one year, abnormal semen parameters if available, or scrotal pain [38].

On the other hand, others found physiological catch up growth at three years on follow up without surgery in boys with original asymmetry 15-20% [39-41].

Although some authors recommend early surgical intervention to preserve fertility, others recommend non operative management based on reported physiological testicular catch up growth during development.

10. Bilaterality

Palpable varicocele is believed to occur on the left side in about 90% of cases while palpable right varicocele is found in 10% of cases of bilateral varicocele [23].

The incidence of subclinical varicocele may be underestimated; the bilaterality of varicocele may be unrecognized if only clinical examination is the only way of diagnosis in the absence of other modalities like; contact thermography, color flow Doppler sonography, and percutaneous retrograde venography to detect subclinical unrecognized right varicocele which is impossible to palpate clinically in more than 90% of cases [42].

Chatel et al noted bilateral varicocele in 60% of 178 patients using thermography; Gonzales et al noted 61% bilateral varicocele using venography [43]. On the other hand, Gat et al using both modalities, noted bilateral varicocele in 85% of patients [44].

This may explain failure of successful unilateral left varicocelectomy alone to restore spermatogenesis in many patients compared to bilateral varicocelectomy as suggested by Scherr and Gold Stien [45].

11. Whom we should repair

It is to be noted that 80-85% of patients with varicocele do not present with infertility, also adolescents with varicocele present only with testicular hypotrophy but not infertility [46].

Varicocelectomy is associated with testicular catch up growth postoperatively but whether early varicocelectomy in boys has a positive effect on future fertility or not, still a matter of discussion [47].

At the same time, catch up growth has been reported in subset of patients with varicocele at three years follow up without surgery.

The indication of varicocelectomy included, asymmetry more than 20%, bad semen parameters if available, pain, and sometimes cosmoses. Till now, no clear guidelines to operate or not to operate on right subclinical varicocele when operating on left clinical varicocele [48].

12. Choice of repair

Management of varicocele includes two categories; percutaneous embolization and surgical treatment. Percutaneous embolization can be done via intravenous injection of occlusive material (sclerotherapy) through retrograde venography. Surgical treatment includes; open varicocelectomy (inguinal, sub inguinal, microscopic sub inguinal) or laparoscopic varicocelectomy. The advantages of embolization include; local anesthesia, low cost, early ambulation, and low complication rates [49].

The failure rate in Ivanissevich repair of adolescent varicocele approached 14-16%, while Kass and Marco reported no failure in 62% Palomo varicocelectomy. The same group reported 3.9% recurrence rate and 29% hydrocele formation incidence in another study included 233 patients [50-52].

Laparoscopic varicocelectomy, sub inguinal lymphatic sparing varicocelectomy were suggested to reduce the incidence of hydrocele [53].

Other group suggested the use of microscope during the Palomo repair to identify lymphatic while others suggested the use of isosulfan blue in this regard [54].

13. Conclusion

Adolescents with varicocele may present at different stages of physical and pubertal development.

There is a need for a guideline for the indications of surgical intervention, type of surgery used, and the ideal protocol for follow up.

http://dx.doi.org/10.5772/59314

Author details

Hosni Khairy Salem

Address all correspondence to: dr_hosni@yahoo.com

Department of Urology, Faculty of Medicine, Cairo University, Egypt

References

[1] TuLLochus: variables in sub fertility; results and treatment, Br Med J1955, 2; 356-358.

[2] Skoog SJ, Roberts KP, Goldstein M, et al. The adolescent varicocele: What's new with an old problem in young patients? Pediatrics, 1997; 100:112-121.

[3] Paduch D, Skoog S. Current management of adolescent's varicocele. Rev Urol.2001; 3:120-133

[4] Raman J, Walmsley K, Goldstien M. Inheritance of varicocele. Adult Urol.2005; 65:1186-1189.

[5] Stavropoulus NE, Mihailidis I, Hastazeris K, et al. Varicocele in school boys. Arch Androl. 2002; 48:187-192.

[6] Akbay E,Cayan S,Doruk E,Duce M,Bozlu M. The prevalence of varicocele- related testicular atrophy in Turkish children and adolescents. BJU.2000; 86:490-493.

[7] Kumanov P, Robeva RN, and Tomova A. Adolescent Varicocele: Who Is at Risk? Pediatrics 2008; 121(1):e35-e57.

[8] World Health Organization: the influence of varicocele on the parameters of infertility in a large group of men presenting with infertility clinics. Fert. Sterl. 1992, 57:1289-1293.

[9] Kass E. The management of the asymptomatic varicocele in adolescence. Probl Urol. 1990; 4:690–704.

[10] Cozzolino DJ, and Lipshultz LI: Varicocele as a progressive lesion: positive effect of varicocele repair. Hum Reprod Update 2001; 7: 55-58.

[11] Pasqualotto FF, Lucon AM, de Goes PM, *et al:* Semen profile, Testicular volume and hormonal levels in infertile patients with Varicoceles compared with fertile men with and without varicoceles. Fertil Steril 2005; 83: 74-77.

[12] Delaney D, Carr M, Kolon T, Snyder H, Zderik S. The physical characteristics of young males with varicocele. BJU.2004; 94:62– 64

[13] Nielsen ME, Zderic S, Freedland SJ, Jarow JP. Insight on pathogenesis of varicocele: relationship of varicocele and body mass index. Urology.2006; 68:392– 396

[14] Handel LN, Shetty R, Sigman M. The relationship between varicoceles and obesity. J Urol.2006; 176:2138– 2140.

[15] Prabakaran S, Kumanov Ph, Tomova A, Hubaveshki S, Agarwal A. Adolescent varicocele: association with somatometric parameters. Urol Int.2006; 77:114– 117

[16] May M, Taymoorian K, Beutner S, et al. Body size and weight as predisposing factors in varicocele. Scand J Urol Nephrol.2006; 40:45– 48

[17] Di Luigi L, Gentile V, Pigozzi F, Parisi A, Gianetti D, Romanelli F. Physical activity as a possible aggravating factor for athletes with varicocele: impact on the semen profile. Hum Reprod.2001; 16:1180– 1184

[18] Di Luigi L, Romanelli F, Pigozzi F, et al. Role of sport medicine in andrological prevention. Med Sport.1994; 47:665– 670.

[19] Paduch D, and Niedzielski J: Repair versus observation in adolescent varicocele: a prospective study. J Urol 158:1128–1132, 1997.

[20] Hamm B, Fobbe F, Sorensen R, *et al:* Varicoceles: combined sonography and thermography in diagnosis and post therapeutic evaluation. Radiology 160: 419–424, 1986.

[21] Chiou KR, Anderson JC, Wobig RK, *et al:* Color Doppler ultrasound criteria to diagnose varicoceles: correlation of a new scoring system with physical examination. Urology 50:953–956, 1997.

[22] Morag B, Rubinstein ZJ, Madgar I, *et al:* The role of spermatic venography after surgical high ligation of the left spermatic veins: diagnosis and percutaneous occlusion. Urol Radiol 7: 32–34, 1985.

[23] Skoog SJ, Roberts KP, Goldstein M, *et al:* The adolescent varicocele: what's new with an old problem in young patients? Pediatrics 100: 112–122, 1997.

[24] Santoro G, Romeo C, Impellizzeri P, et al. Nitric oxide synthase patterns in normal and varicocele testis in adolescent age. Br Urol Int.2001; 88:967– 973.

[25] Sawczuk I, Hensle T, Burbige K, Nagler H. Varicoceles: effect on testicular volume in prepubertal and pubertal males. Urology.1993; 41:466– 468.

[26] Pastuszak AW, Kumar V, Shah A, and Roth D R. Diagnostic and Management Approaches to Pediatric and Adolescent Varicocele: A Survey of Pediatric Urologists; Urology, Articles in press.

[27] Kass EJ, Belman AB: Reversal of testicular growth failure by Varicocele ligation. J Urol 1987, 137:475-6.

[28] Sigman M, Jarow JP: Ipsilateral testicular hypotrophy is associated with decreased sperm counts in infertile men with varicoceles. J Urol 1997, 158:605-7.

[29] Okuyama A, Nakamura M, Namiki M, Takeyama M, Utsunomiya M, Fujioka H, Itatani H, Matsuda M, Matsumoto K, Sonoda T: Surgical repair of varicocele at puberty: preventive treatment for fertility improvement. J Urol 1988, 139:562-4.

[30] Hamm B, Fobbe F, Sorensen R, *et al:* Varicoceles: combined Sonography and thermography in diagnosis and post therapeutic evaluation. Radiology 160: 419–424, 1986.

[31] Chiou KR, Anderson JC, Wobig RK, *et al:* Color Doppler ultrasound criteria to diagnose varicoceles: correlation of a new scoring system with physical examination. Urology 50: 953–956, 1997.

[32] Morag B, Rubinstein ZJ, Madgar I, *et al:* The role of spermatic venography after surgical high ligation of the left spermatic veins: diagnosis and percutaneous occlusion. Urol Radiol 7: 32–34, 1985.

[33] Paduch D, and Niedzielski J: Repair versus observation in adolescent varicocele: a prospective study. J Urol 158: 1128–1132, 1997.

[34] Dubin L, and Amelar RD: Etiologic factors in 1294 consecutive cases of male infertility. Fertil Steril 22: 469–474, 1971.

[35] Kursh ED: What is the incidence of varicocele in a fertile population? Fertil Steril 48: 510–511, 1987.

[36] McClure RD, and Hricak H: Scrotal ultrasound of infertile man: detection of subclinical unilateral and bilateral varicoceles. J Urol 135: 711–715, 1986.

[37] Gonzalez R, Reddy P, Kaye KW, *et al:* Comparison of Doppler examination and retrograde spermatic venography in the diagnosis of varicocele. Fertil Steril 40: 96–99, 1983.

[38] Diamond DA, Zurakowski D, Atala A, et al. Is adolescent varicocele a progressive disease process? J Urol. 2004; 172:1746-1748.

[39] Kolon TF, Clement MR, Cartwright L, et al. Transient asynchronous testicular growth in adolescent males with a varicocele. J Urol. 2008; 180:1111-1114.

[40] Preston MA, Camat T, Flood T, et al. Conservative management of adolescent varicoceles: a retrospective review. Urology. 2008; 72: 77-80.

[41] Poon SA, Gjertson CK, Mercado MA, et al. Testicular asymmetry and adolescent varicoceles managed expectantly. J Urol. 2010; 183: 731-734.

[42] Gorelick JI, and Goldstein M: Loss of infertility in men with varicocele. Fertil Steril 59: 613–616, 1993.

[43] Chatel A, Bigot JM, Helenon C, *et al:* Interet de la phlebographie Spermatique dans le diagnostic das sterilites d'origine circulatory comparison avec les donnes cliniques, thermographiques et anatomiques. Ann Radiol 1978; 21: 565–570.

[44] Gat y, Zukerman z, bachar Gn, feldberg d, and gornish m. adolescent varicocele: is it a unilateral disease? urology2003; 62: 742–747

[45] Scherr D, and Goldstein M: Comparison of bilateral versus unilateral varicolectomy in men with palpable bilateral Varicoceles. J Urol 162: 85–88, 1999.

[46] Pryor JL and Howards SS: Varicocele. Urol Clin North Am 14: 499-513, 1987.

[47] Cozzolino DJ, and Lipshultz LI: Varicocele as a progressive lesion: Positive effect of varicocele repair. Hum Reprod Update 7: 55-58, 2001.

[48] Gorelick JI, and Goldstein M: Loss of fertility in men with varicocele. Fertil Steril 59: 613-616, 1993.

[49] Feber KM, Kass EJ: Varicocelectomy in adolescent boys: long-term experience with the Palomo procedure. J Urol 2008, 180:1657-9; discussion 1659-60

[50] Misseri R, Gershbein AB, Horowitz M, and Glassberg KI: The adolescent Varicocele. II: the incidence of hydrocele and delayed recurrent varicocele after varicocelectomy in a long-term follow-up. BJU Int 2001, 87:494-8.

[51] Kass EJ, Marcol B: Results of varicocele surgery in adolescents: A comparison of techniques. J Urol 1992, 148:694-6.

[52] Feber KM, Kass EJ: Varicocelectomy in adolescent boys: long-term experience with the Palomo procedure. J Urol 2008, 180:1657-9; discussion 1659-60

[53] Glassberg KI, Poon SA, Gjertson CK, DeCastro GJ, Misseri R: Laparoscopic- lymphatic sparing varicocelectomy in adolescents. J Urol 2008, 180:326-30; discussion 330-1

[54] Schwentner C, Oswald J, Lunacek A, Deibl M, Bartsch G, Radmayr C:Optimizing the outcome of microsurgical sub inguinal varicocelectomy using isosulfan blue: a prospective randomized trial. J Urol 2006, 175:1049-52.

Chapter 8

Short-Bowel Syndrome in Children — An Update in Management Strategies

Nick Zavras, Evangelos Misiakos,
Velaoras Konstantinos and Christos Salakos

Additional information is available at the end of the chapter

http://dx.doi.org/10.5772/59313

1. Introduction

Pediatric short bowel syndrome (PSBS) is usually defined as a devastating condition that results from massive intestinal resection due to congenital or acquired lesions and is associated with inadequate absorption of enteral nutrients [1-2]. Additionally, PSBS is accompanied by the loss of the immune capacity and secretion of the intestinal hormones and regulating enteral peptides [3]. Children with PSBS are usually dependent on parenteral nutrition (PN) to compensate fluid, electrolyte and energy requirements [1]. The causes of PSBS vary according to age; in neonates, predominant causes include necrotizing enterocolitis, small bowel atresia and gastroschisis, complicated meconium ileus, and midgut volvulus [4-6]. According to most studies, necrotizing enterocolitis is the most common cause of PSBS in the neonatal period, particularly among extremely premature infants, with an incidence rate ranging from 14% to 43% [4, 7]. In older children, PSBS may be ascribed to Crohn's disease, abdominal tumors, radiation enteritis, trauma, malignancy, iatrogenic lesions and adhesive obstruction [8, 9]. Intestinal motility disorders (total or subtotal aganglionosis) and mucosal enteropathies have also been implicated [10, 11].

There are no accurate data in the literature for the incidence of PSBS [5]; it is based mainly on prematurity and low birth weight [1]. In a large cohort study performed by Cole et al [12], the reported incidence of PSBS among very low birth-weight infants was 0.7% and 1.1% among extremely very low birth-weight infants. Wales et al [13] conducted a retrospective cohort study involving 175 surgical neonates with PSBS, and reported an overall incidence of 22.1/1000 neonatal intensive care unit (NICU) admissions (95% CI=15.3, 28, 9) and 24.8%/

100.000 live births (95% CI=12.1, 36.9). Again, PSBS was higher among premature infants (43.6 of 1000 vs. 3.1 of 1000 admissions).

The mortality rates for PSBS vary extensively between studies and depend on the definitions and causes of PSBS. In general, mortality rates vary from 15% to 40% [13-16]. It is thought that the main risk factors for the high mortality of PSBS include the length of the remaining small bowel, catheter-associated bloodstream infection, loss of ileocecal valve and liver failure due to the prolonged duration of parenteral nutrition [17-21]. Earlier studies concerning PSBS and successful outcome were based on the remaining bowel length after resection and the presence of ileocecal valve (ICV). Wilmore [21] reported a successful outcome of 50% in infants with at least 15cm to 25 cm of residual bowel and an intact ICV, but there were no survivors among those with a residual bowel of 15 cm. However, in a retrospective review of 80 pediatric patients, Spencer et al [22] reported that only cholestasis and the length of the age-adjusted small bowel length can be considered as the strongest predictors of mortality in PSBS. Septic episodes, the presence of ileocecal valve, and the etiology of SBS were not predictive.

The management of PSBS remains a challenge and needs a careful individual curative approach. The aim of the present study is to provide an update of the current therapeutic methods and future aspects in the treatment of PSBS. To this end, PubMed was searched for relevant articles using as key words " short bowel syndrome", "children", "management", "surgical treatment", "medical management", " small bowel transplantation", "tissue engineering", and "experimental approach". The retrieved articles were further screened for additional studies. Articles published in a language other than English were excluded. A brief reference to the pathophysiological changes following intestinal resection is also cited.

1.1. Pathophysiological consequences of PSBS

There are three dominant anatomical anastomoses depending on the extent of the resected bowel: 1) jejunoileal anastomosis, 2) the jejunocolic anastomosis, and 3) end-jejunostomy [23]. Patients of the first group rarely display considerable electrolyte or nutrient imbalance because the residual ileum and the intact colon can balance the absence of the resected bowel [23], due to a) the presence of the less permeable tight junction of the ileum [9] and b) the capacity of the colon for fluid absorption [24]. However, partial resection of the jejunum may impair the secretion of the regulatory hormones produced by jejunal cells. Loss of cholecystokinin released with secretin when food from the stomach reaches the first part of the duodenum may lead to gastric acid hypersecretion due to abolition of the feedback inhibition mechanism that regulates gastrin and gastric acid secretion. This discrepancy may cause an increase in the pH of the proximal small bowel that leads to denature of the pancreatic enzymes and impairment of digestion [25-27]. Experimental studies have shown that patients with jejunocolic anastomosis have more severe disease because the jejunum has reduced adaptive ability as compared to the ileum [28, 29]. Usually, the ICV has also been resected in such cases. The following alterations in the absorption, secretion of fluids, bile salts, lipids and adaption in hormonal mediators due to resection of the ileum may be seen: a) extensive diarrhea due to decreased

http://dx.doi.org/10.5772/59313

water reabsorption by the distal small intestine [9], b) malabsorption of vitamin B_{12} because of the deficiency of receptors of B_{12} localized to the distal ileum [30], c) reduced absorption of bile salts, which in turn may lead to deficiency in fat-soluble vitamins, steatorrhea, and diarrhea [9,30,31], d) up-regulation of glucagon-like peptides 1 and 2 and peptide YY, all of which are produced by enteroendocrine L cells of the distal ileum and colon of patients with ileum resection but with a preserved colon [32, 33]. The net result leads to normal gastric emptying and intestinal transit time for solid foods, less gastric hypersecretion and increase in villus height, crypt cell proliferation, and inhibition of enterocyte apoptosis [23, 34-39]. The loss of both ileum and colon in patients undergoing end-jejunostomy leads to severe dehydration, and electrolyte depletion [23]. Additionally, colon resection results in further depletion of energy as studies have shown that the colon can absorb up to 15% of energy requirements [40-41]. Furthermore, patients with end-jejunostomy display increased gastric emptying and intestinal transportation [42] due to the lack of the protective effect of hormonal mediators such as GLP-1 GLP-2, and peptide YY [23]. Studies in adults have shown that the presence of little or no colon and less than 50-100 cm of jejunum results in permanent parenteral nutrition [43, 44]. However, the results are inconclusive for infants and children, and it seems that colon loss is not a strong predictor for weaning off parenteral nutrition [22, 45, 46].

1.2. Management of PSBS

The current management of patients is multifaceted and includes surgical modification techniques and medical approaches, which will be discussed below. Tissue engineering is also reviewed; this novel strategy, currently in its exploratory phase, aims to build a new small bowel [47].

2. Surgical techniques to treat PSBS

A substantial number of surgical techniques have been described in order to address the two main problems of PSBS: the loss in absorptive surface and dysmotility of the residual above the anastomosis. These procedures pertain to autologous methods of intestinal reconstruction and could be categorized further into two subgroups: I) lengthening of the residual short bowel to provide satisfactory nutrient amount [48,49], and II) slowing of the intestinal transit [4]. Small bowel transplantation represents a separate option and has been proposed as an alternative for children with permanent intestinal failure and no longer tolerated parenteral nutrition (PN) [11, 50].

2.1. Surgical techniques for lengthening of the residual short bowel

a. *Bianchi's procedure.* In 1980, Bianchi was the first to apply the longitudinal intestinal lengthening and tailoring (LILT) technique in an animal model [48]. In brief, this technique consists of a construction from a segment of small intestine of two isoperistaltic hemiloops of half the original diameter. The two hemiloops are then positioned in a circular manner, and an end-to-end anastomosis is performed between them. Subsequently, the new segment is reconnected with the remaining bowel. This allows the doubling of the entire length of the original segment to be performed. Data from the literature suggest that successful outcome is achieved when the following anatomical conditions are met [7]: a) an intestinal diameter > 3 cm; b) a residual small bowel length > 40cm, and c) a dilated bowel length > 20 cm. However, another study by Bianchi [51] of 20 children (aged 7 weeks to 92 months) undergoing LILT, suggested that the favorable outcome (9/20 survivors, 45%) was associated with the presence of >40cm of the residual dilated small intestine and minor hepatic dysfunction. Age, the presence of ICV and the length of the residual colon did not affect survival. In conclusion, LILT seems to increase the function of the residual small bowel; survival rates reach as high as 100% (range 30% to 100%), improvement is noted in intestinal transit, stool frequency, intestinal absorption, weight gain and, in 50% of cases, weaning off parenteral nutrition is observed [51, 52-56].

b. *Kim's procedure.* Serial transverse enteroplasty (STEP) was introduced by Kim et al [49] in 2003 in an experimental study. The technique was performed using a GIA stapler to create a zig-zag channel with a diameter of 2-2.5cm at the mesenteric site. The staples were placed from the 90° and 270° positions at the mesenteric site of the intestine, using the mesentery as the 0° reference point. The basic results showed that the technique is easy to perform, avoids anastomoses, carries a low risk of intestinal ischemia, can be used repeatedly, and could almost double the length of the residual intestine [1].

Recently, Frongia et al [57] compared the above mentioned lengthening techniques in a systematic review. After analyzing the results of 39 articles (LILT: 24, STEP: 15) including 472 patients (LILT: 363 patients, STEP: 109 patients), they concluded that both methods are thought to be acceptable. However, STEP seemed to have a more favourable outcome : LILT 30.2% mortality rate vs. STEP 14.3%. Similar results were reported in a retrospective study by Jones et al [58] who pooled data from the International STEP Data Registry involving the long-term follow-up of 97 patients, aged 2.4 months to 37.8 months, who had undergone STEP. An overall mortality of 11% was recorded. More recently, at small cohort study of 12 children (aged 0.9 to 19 months) was conducted by Wester et al [59]; a t median follow-up of 37.2 (3.0 to 87.5) months, no deaths were recorded.

c. *Cherni's procedure (experimental).* Recently, Cherni et al [60] used a new technique called spiral intestinal lengthening and tailoring (SILT), as an alternative method to LILT and STEP. In brief, spiral incision lines are drawn with a sterile pen to the longitudinal axis of the dilated bowel segment at 45° to 60°. The dilated bowel is then incised along the marks, and the bowel is stretched longitudinally and sutured along the incision line. The purpose of this technique was to minimize injury of the vascular supply of the intestine, as could occur with the LILT procedure, and preserve the anatomy of circular and longitudinal muscle fibers which could be destroyed by the stapler in the STEP technique [59]. The first histopathological results were promising and showed no signs of ischemia and collagen accumulation, while the myenteric, mucosal plexuses and Cajal cell network were normal.

2.2. Surgical techniques to slowing the intestinal transit

a. *Anti-peristaltic segments.* Surgical reconstruction of the residual small bowel using anti-peristaltic jejunal segments has been recommended for patients with a resected ileum and ICV [61]. In summary, the technique includes excision of a small segment (10-15cm in length for adults and 3cm for children) of the distal intestine with its mesenteric blood supply rotation over 180° degree of the distal intestine, and an end-to-end anastomosis between the reversed intestinal segment and the proximal jejunum and distally to the remaining colon [61]. Although, studies in adults [62,63] have shown beneficial results regarding an increase in absorption and weaning from PN, the procedure may be ineffective in the case of an insufficient length of the reversed segment [64]

b. *Colon interposition.* This surgical technique has been used as an adjuvant method in cases of medical management failure. Studies in adults have shown that after interposition, the colon behaves in a similar way to the reversed small intestinal segement [4]. The technique may be performed iso-or antiperistatically [65]. Glick et al [66] used an isoperistaltic colon interposition in six infants with PSBS refractory to medical management. The authors reported a reasonable survival rate of 50% and weaning off total PN. However, this surgical option needs additional studies with a large number of patients to support its effectiveness.

c. *Intestinal valves.* Based on the observed importance of the ICV in the outcome of children with PSBS [21], various techniques have been described for the construction of similar valves. The simplest techniques include the installation of sutures or external Teflon around the circumference of the bowel [67]. Another option involves the creation of small intussusceptions by everting a segment of small bowel [68]. Georgeson et al [69] reported a series of six children in whom a small nipple valve was initially created to provide temporary partial obstruction and thereby induce dilatation and lengthening of the proximal small intestine. In a second stage, they performed an intestinal lengthening procedure. Several of these patients improved and weaned off PN. However, clinical experience of this technique is limited, and the results are based on small series.

d. *Recirculating loops.* Few discouraging results including increased morbidity and mortality have been reported in the literature concerning the use of recirculation loops in the management of PSBS [69]. In addition, improvement of absorption was limited [68].

e. *Tapering enteroplasty.* Tapering enteroplasty is another option in the management of PSBS and involves reducing the caliber of the dilated intestinal segment in patients with PSBS. Usually, this portion exhibits low contraction resulting in stasis, malabsorption and bacterial overgrowth [68]. As patients with PSBS have a short residual intestine, excision of the dilated intestine may be not reasonable. The reduction could be performed either by excising the antimesenteric portion of the dilated segment or by the folding and placation of the intestine [67]. Thomson et al [70] reported a large series of 160 patients including 11 children, aged 6 months to 9 years. All these children had dilated intestinal segments and residual bowel length no longer than 30 cm. Successful enteroplasty with complete weaning from PN was reported in nine (81.8%) children. A drawback to this method is the possible breakdown of the sutures lines with recurrence of dilation and functional obstruction of the bowel [68].

2.3. Intestinal transplantation

Small bowel transplantation is considered the definitive treatment in the management of PSBS. It is indicated in patients with failure of intestinal improvement after various surgical techniques, and in those with no possible feeding tolerance, irreversible hepato-intestinal disease, recurrent sepsis, and failure of their central venous sites [1]. In neonates and small children, liver-intestine or multivisceral transplantation (stomach, pancreaticoduodenal complex, and small intestine) are the choice of treatment [1]. In older children, isolated intestinal transplantation may be used as a further option [1, 11]. Rayes et al reported a one-year patient survival rate of 70% and graft survival rate of 65% [71]. More recently, Lao et al [72] studied the outcome of 852 patients (aged from 1 to 21 years) who had undergone intestinal and/or liver transplantation for short bowel syndrome for various reasons including gastroschisis, necrotizing enterocolitis, volvulus, and others. They found that the relative risk ratio for death was higher among the necrotizing enterocolitis group (p:0.015), lower in those with PSBS for atresias, inflammatory bowel diseases, arterial or venous thrombosis (p:0.001), and not statistically significant in the volvulus group (p:0.094). The authors concluded that underlying disease may influence the outcome of patients. Complications include acute cellular rejection (fever, nausea, vomiting, abdominal distention), graft vs. host disease, and post-transplant lymphoproliferation disorder [11]. The introduction of novel immunosuppressive agents may further improve the outcomes of intestinal transplantation.

3. Medical enhancement of intestinal function

Several peptides, hormones and growth factors have been studied in animal models of SBS the last 20 years. However, few have been investigated in adult patients, and hardly any in children. The most common agents used to alter nutrient absorption will be discussed briefly.

3.1. Epidermal growth factor (EGF)

EGF is a low-molecular-weight polypeptide which enhances cellular proliferation, differentiation, and survival [73]. Sham et al in an experimental study showed that EGF improves carbohydrate absorption and intestinal permeability and reduces weight loss [74]. Possible mechanisms of action include a reduction in apoptosis of intestinal cells, increased expression of the anti-apoptotic gene bcl-w, and decreased expression of the pro-apoptotic gene bax [75]. Several authors have investigated the synergistic role of EGF in experimental studies along with other factors such as interleukin-11, bombesin and neurotensin, and found that they further enhance the adaptive action of EGF [76-78]. Promising results with the use of EGF were reported in a pilot study by Sigalet et al [79] who investigated the effect of enterally administered recombined EGF on nutrient absorption and tolerance feeding in infants with severe PSBS (<25% bowel length for predicting age). EGF was given orally with foods in a daily dose of 100 μg/kg for six weeks The results showed improvement in nutrient absorption, increased tolerance with enteral feeding and possible improvement of infection rate. In contrast, Lukish et al failed to observe any changes in the small bowel epithelium after an experimental massive intestinal resection and utilization of EGF [80].

3.2. Growth hormone (GH)

GH is a single chain protein comprising 191 amino-acids and is produced in the pituitary gland [81]. Receptors of GH have been found throughout the intestine, including muscularis propria, submucosa muscularis, lamina propria, muscularis mucosa and intestinal epithelium [82]. Laboratory studies have shown that GH causes mucosal hyperplasia and increases the adaptive capacity after small resection [83, 84]. Other actions of GH include enhancement of the villus height and crypt depth, positive nitrogen balance and bowel growth when rats were given GH combined with glutamine and/or a diet high in protein [85,86].Studies in children with PSBS showed a reduction in PN [87], but after cessation of GH the positive response could not be preserved [88)]. The results in adults are controversial. For example, Scolapio et al [89] reported no benefits from the administration of recombinant human GH (rhGH) in adult patients with SBS. On the contrary, Seguy et al [90] showed a significant increase in absorption rates, followed by a decrease in PN requirements.

3.3. Glucagon-Like Peptide 2 (GLP-2)

GLP-2 is a 33-amino acid peptide that is secreted by enteroendocrine L-cells which are found mainly in the terminal ileum and colon (91. Release of GLP-2 is stimulated by food input, directly or indirectly promoting intestinal growth and nutrient absorption [91, 92]. Patients who had undergone ileal resection and jejunostomy have a diminished secretion of GLP-2 [93], while those submitted to ileal resection but with preservation of colon in continuity have elevated levels of GLP-2 at baseline, compared with the control group, which remain high following a meal [32]. Teleglutide is an analog of GLP-2 with a longer half-life which encourages villus height and increases crypt depth, improving nutrient absorption, gastric emptying and body weight [94]. Using an animal model with preterm pigs, Vegge et al [95] recently showed that GLP-2 enhances rapid digestion adaption and improves digestion function in preterm pigs with jejunostomy.

3.4. Insulin-like Growth Factor-1 (IGF-1)

IGF-1 is secreted primarily by hepatocytes, and activated by GH [96]. A review of Bordvedt et al [97] provided strong evidence that IGF-1 mediates growth effects of GH and GLP-2 on the intestine or continuous growth in experimental models of bowel resection or Crohn's disease, besides the perception that these hormones or IGF-1 may reinforce further growth if given shortly after bowel resection. Similarly, using a rat model, Chen et al [98] demonstrated that IGF-1 may prevent mucosal atrophy, enhance gut metabolism, and protect the intestinal barrier against sepsis. Furthermore, Barksdale et al [99] showed that children with PSBS demonstrated growth failure despite adequate nutritional support. Serological tests for GH,

IGF-1, and thyroid function showed that only IGF-1 and IGFPB-3 correlated with growth failure.

3.5. Hepatocyte Growth-Factor (HGF)

HGF is secreted by mesenchymal cells and carries trophic properties [96]. Laboratory studies have demonstrated that HGF enhances small intestine growth and absorptive function regarding carbohydrates and amino-acids. However, there are no clinical data on human beings.

4. Tissue Engineering Small Intestine (TESI)

TESI comprises a new complex field in the management of PSBS. In order to build a viable and functional small intestine, the armamentarium of TESI includes sophisticated materials, human pluripotential stem cells, and biopharmaceutical means [100].

Salerno-Gonsalves et al [101] designed an organotypic model consisting of fibroblasts, lymphocytes, epithelial and endothelial cells, in order to create a comparable and functional structure to human intestinal mucosa. Their concept based on previous observations showed that the culture of endothelial and epithelial cells under microgravity could self-organize into structures resembling native tissues. [102-105]. Although their results showed differentiated cell-types and villus-like structures, the mesenchyma was absent.

Human pluripotent cells [both embryonic and induced pluripotent stem cells], in vitro, have been shown to differentiate in tissues resembling those of the fetal bowel with secretory and absorptive properties [106]. Although these mesenchymal markers detected the presence of a mesenchymal layer, the structures lacked blood vessels and nerves; hence, these strategies could not be used for correct growth of a full thickness intestine.

Promising results may derive from plugs of full thickness intestine called organoid units. Studies have shown that organoid units, placed on a coated scaffold implanted in the omentum of rats, acquired vessels and developed a cyst-shaped structure resembling a small intestine [107]. After placement in continuity with the small intestine, rats returned to their preoperative weight [108, 109].

A number of proteins or nucleic acid, known as biopharmaceuticals, have been used either in clinical trials or in vitro [110]. Available biopharmaceuticals products include IGF-I, IGF-II, EGF, TNF-a, etc. However, a substantial number of these products are currently not used in clinical practice or in TESI.

5. Conclusion

The management strategies of PSBS have expanded over the last 20 years. New surgical techniques and innovative medical and nutritional inventions are used to improve survival

http://dx.doi.org/10.5772/59313

and quality of life in patients with PSBS. Research of new fields, such as TESI and biopharmaceutical agents, could lead to a more successful and definite treatment of PSBS.

Author details

Nick Zavras[1], Evangelos Misiakos[1], Velaoras Konstantinos[2] and Christos Salakos[3]

1 3rd Department of General Surgery, University Hospital "Attikon", Athens, Greece

2 Department of Pediatric Surgery, Penteli General Children's Hospital, Athens, Greece

3 Department of Pediatric Surgery, University Hospital "Attikon", Athens, Greece

References

[1] Sulkowski JP, Minneci PC. Management of short bowel syndrome. Pathophysiology 2014; 21: 111-118

[2] Kokoshis SA. Medical management of pediatric intestinal failure. Semin Pediatr Surg 2010; 19: 20-26

[3] Tumas R, Zamberlan P, Cardoso AL. Use of symbiotic supplement in a child with short bowel syndrome; a case report. Nutr Hosp 2014; 29: 215-220

[4] Welh S, Kessler M. Fononni H, Golriz M, Hafezi M, Mehrabi A, Holland-Cunz S. Current practice and future perspectives in the treatment of short bowel syndrome in children-a systematic review. Langenbecks Arch Surg 2012; 197: 1043-1051

[5] Wales PW, Christison-Lagay ER. Short bowel syndrome: epidemiology and etiology. Semin Pediatr Surg 2010; 19: 3-9

[6] Spencer AU, Kovasevich D, McKinney-Barnet M...Pediatric short-bowel syndrome: the cost of comprehensive care. Am J Clin Nutr 2008; 88: 1552-1559

[7] Goulet O, Sauvat F. Short bowel syndrome and intestinal transplantation in children. Curr Opin Clin Nutr Metab Care 2006; 9: 304-313

[8] DiBaise JK, Young RJ, Vanderhoof JA. Intestinal rehabilitation and the short bowel syndrome. Am J Gastroelnterol 2004;99: 1386-1395

[9] Hölwarth ME. Short bowel syndrome: pathological and clinical aspects. Pathophysiology 1999; 6: 1-19

[10] Schulzje JD, Troger H, Amashch M. Disorders of intestinal secretion and absorption. Best Pract Res Clin Gastroenterol 2009; 23: 395-406

[11] Yildiz BD. Where are we at with short bowel syndrome and small bowel transplant? World J Transplant 2012; 2: 95-103

[12] Cole CR, Hansen NI, Higgins RD. Very low birth weight preterm infants with surgical short bowel syndrome: incidence, morbidity and mortality, and growth outcomes at 18 to 22 months. Pediatrics 2008; 122: e573-e582

[13] Wales PW, de Silva N, Kim J, Lecce L, To T, Moore A. Neonatal short bowel syndrome: population-based estimates of incidence and mortality rates. J Pediatr Surg 2004; 39: 690-695

[14] Quirós-Tejeira RE, Ament ME, Reyen L, Herzog F, Merjanian M, Olivares-Serrano N, Vargas JH. Long-term parenteral nutritional support and intestinal adaptation in children with short bowel syndrome: a 25-year experience. J Pediatr 2004; 145: 157-163

[15] Wales PW, de Silva N, Kim JH, Lecce L, Sandhu A, Moore AM. Neonatal short bowel syndrome: a cohort study. J Pediatr Surg 2005: 40:755-762

[16] Grosfeld JL, Rescolta FJ, West KW. Short bowel syndrome in infancy and childhood. Analysis of survival in 60 patients. Am J Surg 1986; 151: 41-46

[17] Bueno J, Guiterrez J, Mazariegos GV, Abu-Elmagd K, Madariaga J, Ohwada S,Kocoshis S, Reyes J. Analysis of patients with longitudinal intestinal lengthening procedure referred to intestinal transplantation. J Pediatr Surg 2001; 36: 178-183

[18] Vanderhoof JA, Langnas AN. Short bowel syndrome in children and adults. Gastroenterology 1997; 113: 1767-1778

[19] Ziegler MM. Short bowel syndrome: remedial features that influence outcome nd duration of parenteral nutrition. J Pediatr 1997; 131: 335-336

[20] Teiterlbaum DH. Parenteral nutrition-associated cholestasis. Curr Opin Pediatr 1997; 9: 270-275

[21] Wilmore DW. Factors correlating with a successful outcome following extensive intestinal resection in newborn infants. J Pediatr 1972; 80:88-95

[22] Spencer AU, Neaga A, West B, Safran J, Brown P, Btaiche I. Kuzma-O'Reilly B, Teitelbaum DH. Pedaitric short bowel syndrome: redefining predictors of success. Ann Surg 2005; 242: 403-412

[23] Tappenden KA. Pathophysiology of short bowel syndrome: considerations of resected and residual anatomy. J Parenteral Ent N 2014; 20:1-9

[24] Debongnic JC, Philips SF. Capacity of the human colon to absorb fluid. Gastroenterology 1978; 74: 751-756

[25] Sundaram A, Koutkia P, Apovian CM. Nutritional management of short bowel syndrome in adults. J Clin Gastroenterol 2002; 34: 207-220

http://dx.doi.org/10.5772/59313

[26] Jin HO, Lee KY, Chang TM, Chey WY, Dubois A. Secretin: a physiological regulator of gastric emptying and acid output in dogs. Am J Physiol 1994; 267: G702-G708

[27] Nightingale J, Spiller R. Normal intestinal anatomy and physiology. In: Nightingale JDM, ed. Intestinal failure. London UK: Greenwich Medical Media; 2001: 15-36

[28] Dowling RH, Booth CC. Structural and functional changes following small intestinal resection in the rat. Clin Sci 1967; 32: 139-149

[29] Thompson JS, Quigley EM, Adrian TE. Factors affecting outcome following proximal and distal intestinal resection in the dog: an examination of the relative roles of mucosal adaption, motility luminal factors, and enteric peptides. Dig Dis Sci 1999;44: 63-74

[30] Matarese LE. Nutrition and fluid optimization for patients with short bowel syndrome. JPEN J Parenter Enteral Nutr 2013; 37 161-170

[31] Eusufzai S. Bile acid malabsorption: mechanisms and treatment. Dig Dis 1995; 13: 312-321

[32] Jeppesen PB, Hartmann B, Thulesen J, Hansen B S, Holst J J, Poulsen S S, Mortensen P B. Elevated plasma glucagon-like peptide 1 and 2 concentrations in ileum resected short bowel patients with a preserved colon. Gut 2000; 47: 370-376

[33] Nightgale JM, Kamm MA, van der Sijp JR, Ghatei MA, Bloom SR, Lennard-Jones JE. Gastroinestinal hormones in short bowel syndrome. Peptide YY may be the "colonic brake" to gastric emptying. Gut 1996; 39: 267-272

[34] Landor JH, Behringer BR, Wild RA. Postenterectomy gastric hypersecretion in dogs: the relative importance of proximal versus distal resection. J Surg Res1971;11:238-242

[35] Nightingale JM, Lennard-Jones JE. The short bowel syndrome: what's new and old? Dig Dis. 1993;11:12-31

[36] Jeppesen PB, Sanguinetti EL, Buchman A, Howard L, Scolapio JS, Ziegler TR,Gregory J, Tappenden KA, Holst J, Mortensen PB. Teduglutide (ALX-0600), a dipeptidyl peptidase IV resistant glucagon-like peptide 2 analogue, improves intestinal function in short bowel syndrome patients. Gut 2005 Sep;54:1224-1231

[37] Jeppesen PB, Hartmann B, Thulesen J, Graff J, Lohmann J, Hansen BS, Tofteng F, Poulsen SS, Madsen JL, Holst JJ, Mortensen PB. Glucagon-like peptide 2 improves nutrient absorption and nutritional status in short-bowel patients with no colon. Gastroenterology 2001; 120:806-815

[38] Drucker DJ, Erlich P, Asa SL, Brubaker PL. Induction of epithelial cell proliferation by glucagon-peptide 2. Proc Natl Acad Sci USA 1996; 93: 7911-7916

[39] Tappenden KA, Edelman J, Joelsson B. Teduglutide enhances structural adaptation of the small intestinal mucosa in patients with short bowel syndrome. J Clin Gastroenterol 2013 ;47:602-607

[40] Nordgaard I, Hansen BS, Mortensen PB. Colon as a digestive organ in patients with short bowel. Lancet 1994; 343: 373-376

[41] Jeppesen PB, Mortensen PB. Significance of a preserved colon for parenteral energy requirements in patients receiving home parenteral nutrition. Scand J Gastroenterol 1998; 33:1175-1179

[42] Little TJ, Doran S, Meyer JH, Smout AJ, O'Donovan DG, Wu KL, Jones KL, Wishart J, Rayner CK, Horowitz M, Feinle-Bisset C. The release of GLP-1 and ghrelin, but not GIP and CCK, by glucose is dependent upon the length of small intestine exposed. Am J Physiol Endocrinol Metab 2006 ;291:E647-E655

[43] Jeong SH, Lee HJ, Bae HJ, Kim Y, Yoo MW, Yoon YK, Yang HK. Factors affecting postoperative dietary adaptation in short bowel syndrome. Hepatogastroenterology 2009 Jul-Aug;5693:1049-1052

[44] Gouttebel MC, Saint-Aubert B, Astre C, Joyeux H. Total parenteral nutrition needs in different types of short bowel syndrome. Dig Dis Sci 1986;31:718-723

[45] Kaufman SS, Loseke CA, Lupo JV, Young RJ, Murray ND, Pinch LW, Vanderhoof JA. Influence of bacterial overgrowth and intestinal inflammation on duration of parenteral nutrition in children with short bowel syndrome. J Pediatr 1997 ;131:356-361

[46] Diamond IR, Struijs MC, de Silva NT, Wales PW. Does the colon play a role in intestinal adaptation in infants with short bowel syndrome? A multiple variable analysis. J Pediatr Surg. 2010;45:975-979

[47] Belchior GG, Sogayar MC, Grikscheit TC. Stem cells and biopharmaceuticals: vital roles in the growth of tissue-engineered small intestine Semin Pediatr Surg. 2014 ; 23:141-149

[48] Bianchi A. Intestinal loop lengthening-A technique for increasing small bowel length. J Pediatr Surg 1980; 15: 145-151

[49] Kim HB, Garza D, Oh J-T, Nurko S, Jaksic T. Serial transverse enteroplasty (STEP); A novel bowel lengthening procedure. J Pediatr Surg 2003: 38: 425-428

[50] Jayarajn S, Daller JA. Reverse intestinal interposition: a model for living related transplantation? J Surg Res 2011; 169: 192-193

[51] Bianchi A. Longitudinal intestinal lengthening and tailoring: results in 20 children. J R Soc Med 1997; 90:429-432

[52] Ching YA, Gura K, Modi B, Jacsic T. Pediatric intestinal failure: nutrition, pharmacologic, and surgical approach. Nutr Clin Pract 2007; 22: 654-663

[53] Bianchi A. From the cradle to enteral autonomy: the role of autologous gastrointestinal reconstruction. Gastroenterology 2006; 130 (2 Suppl):S138-S146

[54] Georgeson K, Halpin D, Figueroa R, Vincente Y, Hardin W Jr. Sequential intestinal lengthening for refractory short bowel syndrome. J Pediatr Surg 1994; 29: 316-320

[55] Weber TR. Isoperistaltic bowel lengthening for short bowel syndrome in children. Am J Surg 1999; 178: 600-604

[56] Boeckman CR, Traylor B. Bowel lengthening for short gut syndrome. J Pediatr Surg 1981; 16: 996-997

[57] Frongia G, Kessler M, Weih S, Nickkolgh A, Mehrabi A, Holland-Cuz S. Comparison of LILT and STEP procedures in children with short bowel syndrome-A systematic review of the literature. J Pediatr Surg 2013: 48; 1794-1805

[58] Jones BA, Hull MA, Potanos KM, Zurakowski D, Firzgibbons SC, Ching YA, Duggan C, Jaksic T, Kim HR. Report of 111 consecutive patients enrolled in the International Serial Transverse Enteroplasty (STEP) Data Registry. J Am Coll Surg 2013; 216:438-446

[59] Wester T, Borg H, Naji H, Stenström G, Westbacke G, Lilja HE. Serial transverse enteroplasty to facilitate enteral autonomy in selected patients with short bowel syndrome. Br J Surg 2014; 101: 1329-1333

[60] Cherni T, Varga G, Ercs D, Kaszaki J, Boros N, Lazlo A, Murphy F, Földvari A, Morabito A, Bianchi A, Rakoczy G. Spiral intestinal lengthening and tailoring-first in vivo sudy. J Pediatr Surg 2013; 48: 1907-1913

[61] Thomson JS, Rikkers LF. Surgical attempts for the short bowel syndrome. Am J Gastroenterol 1987; 82: 97-106

[62] Pigot F, Messing B, Chaussade S, Pfeiifer A, Pouliquen X, Jian R. Severe short bowel syndrome with a surgically reversed small bowel segment. Dig Dis Sci 1990; 35: 137-144

[63] Panis Y, Messing B, Rivet P, Coffin B, Hautefeuille P, Matuchansky C, Rambaud JC, Valleur P. Segmental reversal of the small bowel as an alternative to intestinal transplantation in patients with short bowel syndrome. Ann Surg 1997; 225:401-407

[64] Bianchi A. Form the cradle to enteral autonomy: the role of autologous gastrointestinal reconstruction. Gastroenterology 2006; 30: S138-S148

[65] Thompson JS. Surgical therapy for the short bowel syndrome. J Surg Res 1985; 39: 81-91

[66] Glick PL, de Lorimier AA, Adzick NS, Harrison MR. Colon interposition: an adjuvant operation for short-gut syndrome. J Pediatr Surg. 1984;19:719-725

[67] Stahlgern LH, Roy RH, Umana G. A mechanical impediment in intestinal fow: Physiological effects on intestinal absorption. JAMA 1964; 187: 41-44

[68] Warner BW. Sort-Bowel syndrome. In: Pediatric Surgery, vol II. Grosfeld JL, O'Neil JA Jr, Fonkalsrud EW, Coran AG (eds). Philadelphia, Mosby 2006: 1369-1382

[69] Georgeson K, Halpin D, Figueroa R, Vincente Y, Hardin W Jr. Sequential intestinal lengthening procedures for refractory short bowel syndrome. J Pediatr Surg. 1994;2:316-320; discussion 320-321

[70] Thompson JS, Langnas AN, Pinch LW, Kaufman S, Quigley EM, Vanderhoof JA. Surgical approach to short-bowel syndrome. Experience in a population of 160 patients. Ann Surg. 1995 ;222:600-605

[71] Rayes J. Intestinal transplantation for children with short bowel syndrome. Semin Pediatr Surg 2001; 10:99-104

[72] Lao OB, Healey PJ, Perkins JD, Horslen S, Reyes JD, Goldin AB. Outcomes in children after intestinal transplant. Pediatrics. 2010 ;125:e550-e558

[73] Herbst RS.Review of epidermal growth factor receptor biology". Int J Radiol Oncol Biol Phys 2004; 59 (2 Suppl): 21–26

[74] Sham J, Martin G, Meddings JB, Sigalet DL. Epidermal growth factor improves nutritional outcome in a rat model of short bowel syndrome. J Pediatr Surg 2002;37:765-769

[75] Stern LE, Falcone RA, Huang F, Kemp CJ, Erwin CR, Warner BW. Epidermal growth factor alters the bax:bcl-w ratio following massive small bowel resection. J Surg Res. 2000;911:38–42

[76] Fiore NF, Ledniczky G, Liu Q, Orazi A, Du X, Williams DA, Grosfeld JL. Comparison of interleukin-11 and epidermal growth factor on residual small intestine after massive small bowel resection. J Pediatr Surg 1998; 33:24–29

[77] Iskit SH, Tugtepe H, Ayyildiz SH, Kotiloglu E, Dagli TE, Yeğen BC. Epidermal growth factor and bombesin act synergistically to support intestinal adaptation in rats with massive small bowel resection. Pediatr Surg Int 2005; 21 :436–440

[78] Ryan CK, Miller JH, Seydel AS, de Mesy Jensen K, Sax HC. Epidermal growth factor and neurotensin induce microvillus hypertrophy following massive enterectomy. J Gastrointest Surg 1997; 1:467–73

[79] Sigalet DL, Martin GR, Butzner JD, Buret A, Meddings JB. A pilot study of the use of epidermal growth factor in pediatric short bowel syndrome. J Pediatr Surg. 2005 May;40: 763-768

[80] Lukish J, Schwartz MZ, Rushin JM, Riordan GP. A comparison of the effect of growth factors on intestinal function and structure in short bowel syndrome. J Pediatr Surg. 1997 ;32:1652-1655

[81] Delehaye-Zervas MC, Mertani H, Martini JF, Nihoul-Feketé C, Morel G,Postel-Vinay MC. Expression of the growth hormone receptor gene in human digestive tissue. J Clin Endocrinol Metab. 1994 Jun;78:1473-1480

[82] Zhou X, Li YX, Li N, Li JS. Glutamine enhances the gut-trophic effect of growth hormone in rat after massive small bowel resection. J Surg Res 2001 Jul;99:47-52

[83] Gu Y, Wu ZH, Xie JX, Jin DY, Zhuo HC. Effects of growth hormone (rhGH) and glutamine supplemented parenteral nutrition on intestinal adaptation in short bowel rats. Clin Nutr. 2001 Apr;20:159-166

[84] Waitzberg DL, Cukier C, Mucerino DR, Logulo AF, Torrinhas RS, de Castro I.Small bowel adaptation with growth hormone and glutamine after massive resection of rat's small bowel. Nutr Hosp. 1999 ;14:81-90

[85] Fadrique B, Lopez JM, Bermudez R, Gomez de Segura IA, Vazquez I, De Miguel E. Growth hormone plus high protein diet promotes adaptation after massive small bowel resection in aged rats. Exp Gerontol 2001;36:1727–1737

[86] Ladd AP, Grosfeld JL, Pescovitz OH, Johnson NB. The effect of growth hormone supplementation on late nutritional independence in pediatric patients with short bowel syndrome. J Pediatr Surg. 2005 ;40:442-425

[87] Goulet O, Dabbas-Tyan M, Talbotec C, Kapel N, Rosilio M, Souberbielle JC, Corriol O, Ricour C, Colomb V. Effect of recombinant human growth hormone on intestinal absorption and body composition in children with short bowel syndrome. JPEN J Parenter Enteral Nutr. 2010 ;34:513-520

[88] McMellen ME, Wakeman D, Longshore SW, McDuffie LA, Warner BW. Growth factors: possible roles for clinical management of the short bowel syndrome. Semin Pediatr Surg 2010;19:35-43

[89] Scolapio JS, Camilleri M, Fleming CR, Oenning LV, Burton DD, Sebo TJ, Batts KP, Kelly DG. Effect of growth hormone, glutamine, and diet on adaptation in short-bowel syndrome: a randomized, controlled study. Gastroenterology. 1997 ; 113:1074-81

[90] Seguy D, Vahedi K, Kapel N, Souberbielle JC, Messing B. Low-dose growth hormone in adult home parenteral nutrition-dependent short bowel syndrome patients: a positive study. Gastroenterology 2003;124:293-302

[91] Peterson J, Kerner JA Jr, New advances in the management of children with intestinal failure. J Parenter Enter Nutr 2012; 36: S36-S42

[92] Estall JL, Drucker DJ. Glucagon-like Peptide-2. Annu Rev Nutr 2006; 26: 391–411

[93] Yusta B, Holland D, Koehler JA, Maziarz M, Estall JL, Higgins R, Drucker DJ. ErbB signaling is required for the proliferative actions of GLP-2 in the murine gut. Gastroenterology 2009; 137: 986–996

[94] Jeppesen PB, Hartmann B, Hansen BS, Thulesen J, Holst JJ, Mortensen PB. Impaired meal stimulated glucagon-like peptide 2 response in ileal resected short bowel patients with intestinal failure. Z MZ. Gut 1999;45:559-653

[95] Vegge A, Thymann T, Lund P, Stoll B, Bering SB, Hartmann B, Jelsing J, Qvist N, Burrin DG, Jeppesen PB, Holst JJ, Sangild PT. Glucagon-like peptide-2 induces rapid digestive adaptation following intestinal resection in preterm neonates. Am J Physiol Gastrointest Liver Physiol 2013 15;305:G277-G285

[96] Schwartz MZ. Novel therapies for the management of short bowel syndrome in children. Pediatr Surg Int 2013; 29: 967-974

[97] Bordvedt SF, Lund PK. Insulin-like growth factor 1: common mediator of multiple enterotrphic hormones and growth factors. Curr Opin Gastroenterol 2012; 28: 89-98

[98] Chen K, Okuma T, Okamura K, Tabira Y, Kaneko H, Miyauchi Y. Insulin-like growth factor-I prevents gut atrophy and maintains intestinal integrity in septic rats. JPEN J Parenter Enteral Nutr 1995;19:119-1124

[99] Barksdale EM Jr, Koehler AN, Yaworski JA, Gardner M, Reyes J. Insulinlike growth factor 1 and insulinlike growth factor 3: indices of intestinal failure in children. J Pediatr Surg 1999 ;34:655-561

[100] Belchior GG, Sogayar MC, Grikscheit TC. Stem cells and biopharmaceuticals: vital roles in the growth of tissue-engineered small intestine. Semin Pediatr Surg 2014;2:141-149

[101] Salerno-Goncalves R, Fasano A, Sztein MB. Engineering of a multicellular organotypic model of the human intestinal mucosa. Gastroenterology 2011;141:e18-20

[102] Carvalho HM, Teel LD, Goping G, O'Brien AD. A three-dimensional tissue culture model for the study of attach and efface lesion formation by enteropathogenic and enterohaemorrhagic Escherichia coli. Cell Microbiol 2005;7:1771–1781

[103] Khaoustov VI, Darlington GJ, Soriano HE, Krishnan B, Risin D, Pellis NR, Yoffe B. Induction of three-dimensional assembly of human liver cells by simulated microgravity. In Vitro Cell Dev Biol Anim 1999;35:501–509

[104] Sanford GL, Ellerson D, Melhado-Gardner C, Sroufe AE, Harris-Hooker S. Three-dimensional growth of endothelial cells in the microgravity-based rotating wall vessel bioreactor. In Vitro Cell Dev Biol Anim 2002;38:493–504

[105] Su GN, Hidaka M, Kimura Y, Yamamoto G. In situ collagen gelation: a new method for constructing large tissue in rotary culture vessels. In Vitro Cell Dev Biol Anim 2003; 39:368–374

[106] Spence JR, Mayhew CN, Rankin SA, Kuhar MF, Vallance JE, Tolle K, Hoskins EE, Kalinichenko VV, Wells SI, Zorn AM, Shroyer NF, Wells JM. Directed differentiation of

human pluripotent stem cells into intestinal tissue in vitro. Nature 2011 ;470(7332): 105-109

[107] Dunn JC. Is the tissue-engineered intestine clinically viable? Nat Clin Pract Gastroenterol Hepatol 2008;5:366-367

[108] Warner BW. Tissue engineered small intestine: a viable clinical option. Ann Surg 2004; 240: 755-756

[109] Grikscheit TC, Siddique A, Ochoa ER, Srinivasan A, Alsberg E, Hodin RA, Vacanti JP. Tissue-engineered small intestine improves recovery after massive small bowel resection. Ann Surg 2004 ;240:748-754

[110] Walsh G. Biopharmaceutical and biotechnology medicines: an issue of nomenclature. Eur J Pharm Sci 2002; 15: 135-138